A GIFT FOR

_____

FROM

_____

DATE

_____

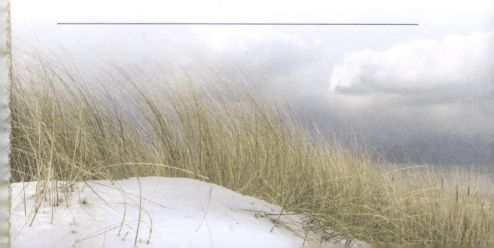

THE
STRESS
LESS

DEVOTIONAL

**100 DAYS
to Embrace Rest and
Rejuvenate Your Soul**

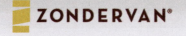

ZONDERVAN

The Stress Less Devotional

Copyright © 2025 by Zondervan

Published in Grand Rapids, Michigan, by Zondervan. Zondervan is a registered trademark of The Zondervan Corporation, L.L.C., a wholly owned subsidiary of HarperCollins Christian Publishing, Inc.

Requests for information should be addressed to customercare@harpercollins.com.

Portions of this book have been previously published in *365 Devotions for Finding Rest* by Christina M. Vinson.

Images used under license from Shutterstock.com.

Art direction and cover design: Sabryna Lugge
Interior design: Kristy Edwards

ISBN 978-0-3104-6686-4 (HC)
ISBN 978-0-310-46687-1 (eBook)

Printed in India

25 26 27 28 29 MAN 10 9 8 7 6 5 4 3 2 1

CONTENTS

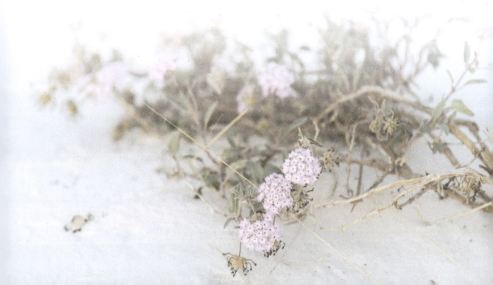

INTRODUCTION

S tress. In today's fast-paced, anxiety-ridden world, everyone's stressed, or so it seems. When was the last time you didn't feel overwhelmed or stretched beyond your limits or, in a word, *stressed*?

How you manage stress makes all the difference in how it affects your life. A little stress isn't bad—it keeps you on your toes as you deal with both your daily activities and any challenges that arise. But an abundance of unchecked stress can cause all sorts of problems—physical, mental, and relational.

If you're searching for a way to break free from this often-crippling burden—if you're looking to satisfy the deep, God-given yearning in your soul for peace and to quiet the buzzing in your mind that comes from too much activity and not enough downtime—this devotional is for you.

In Matthew 11:28–29, Jesus said, "Come to me, all who labor and are heavy laden, and I will give you rest. Take my yoke upon you, and learn from me, for I am gentle and lowly in heart, and you will find rest for your souls" (esv). Doesn't that sound wonderful? Jesus speaks truth—and only truth. When He says He will give you rest, He means it. When He says you will find rest for your stressed-out soul, you will.

So take a deep breath, relax your shoulders, and let your thoughts unwind. Ask the Lord to reveal Himself and His truth to you like never before. And ask Him to show you how to live a restful, stress-free life.

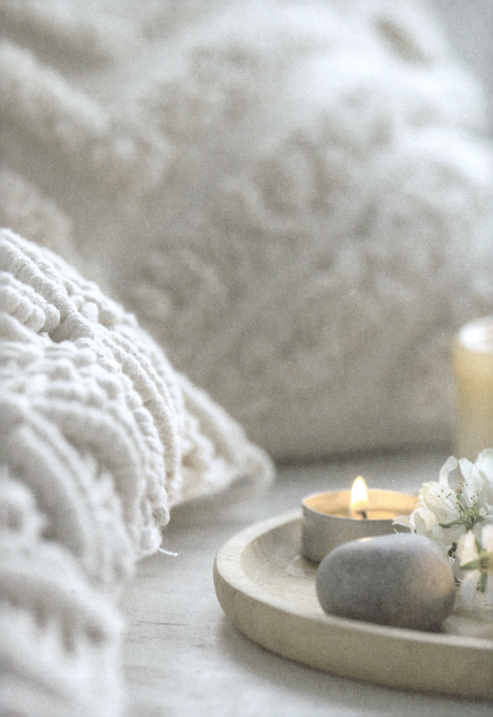

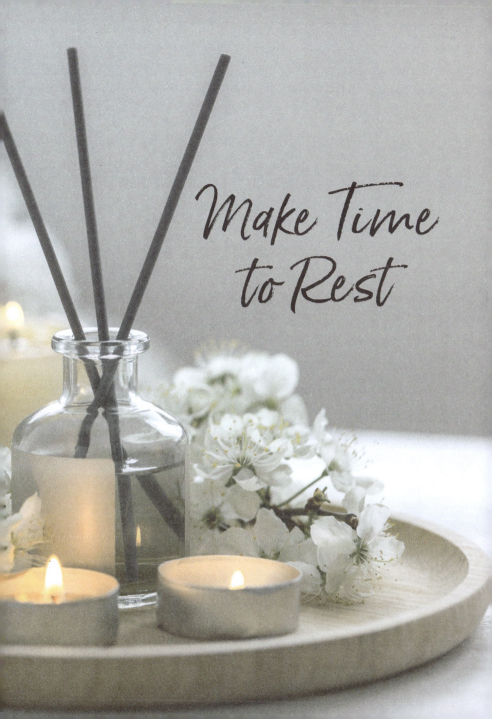

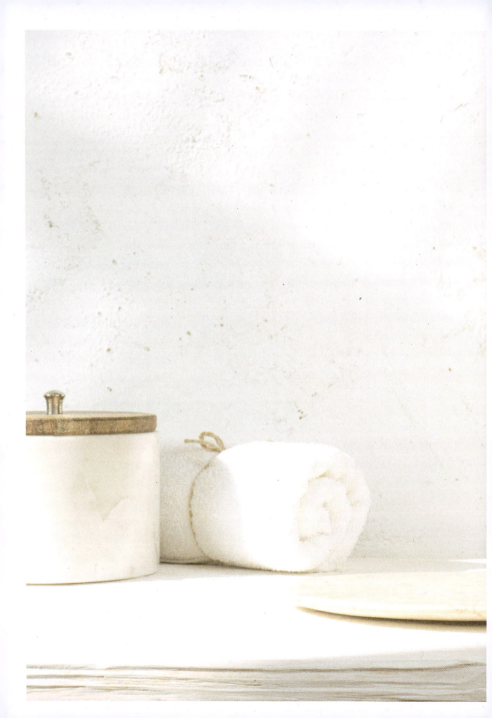

CHOOSE REST OVER STRESS

**In repentance and rest is your salvation, in
quietness and trust is your strength.**
Isaiah 30:15

I'm *so stressed.* How often do we hear—and say—that phrase? But stress isn't good, and it's not something to be proud of. For many of us, though, stressed is our default state of being.

So how do you find relief in a stressed-out culture? You find ways to rest. You choose to spend quiet time with the Lord in the morning, even when every inch of you wants to run around getting ready and checking things off your list. You turn to the Lord when you feel overwhelmed, and you ask a friend for help when you're frazzled.

Simply put, you choose rest. Rest won't just happen; it must be intentionally and deliberately sought out. And to find it, you must ask the Lord to guide you to it. Give all your fears and worries over to Him. Choosing rest means choosing to rely on the Lord—and He will lead you to rest.

*God, when I feel stressed, remind me
that I can choose to rest in You.*

MAKE TIME FOR RETREAT

**Our present sufferings are not worth comparing
with the glory that will be revealed in us.**
Romans 8:18

Quiet. *Solitude. Sleep. Rejuvenation.* Even the words sound wonderful. You may be longing for deep, soul-quieting rest, but the daily demands of your life make it an unlikely dream. Take comfort in these promises from Isaiah: "The LORD is the everlasting God. . . . He will not grow tired or weary. . . . Those who hope in the LORD will renew their strength. They will soar on wings like eagles; they will run and not grow weary, they will walk and not be faint" (Isaiah 40:28, 31).

Not only does the Lord not grow tired or weary, but He also gives you strength when you are weary. Even if you can't escape the busyness of your life, you can still find rest for your soul. Take comfort in the Lord's words today, dear friend. He can give you retreat and reprieve—even in the midst of your rush-and-tumble day. Ask Him for it, then thank Him for the answer you can believe is coming.

Lord, I'm so grateful that You don't grow weary
and that You promise to give me strength.

IS THIS FRUITFUL?

Walk in a manner worthy of the Lord, fully pleasing to him: bearing fruit in every good work and increasing in the knowledge of God.
Colossians 1:10 ESV

As Christians, we feel the call to serve. We serve on committees, as elders and deacons, and as teachers. We visit the elderly, take meals to needy families, and participate in a plethora of other service-related activities. Those are all good things, but just because an opportunity arises doesn't mean you're the one called to do it.

Overcommitment, even to good things, brings additional stress. If you need to cut back, ask yourself, *Is this service fruitful? Is it a good fit for my season of life? Am I serving out of love or obligation?* Those are tough questions, but when life is speeding by at a record pace, you need to ask them.

Asking these questions may bring relief or nervousness. You might even feel guilt or anxiety about taking something off your plate. But remember: Your heavenly Father has the perfect answers. Ask Him to show you where you are needed and where you can step down—and find rest in His answers.

Father, guide my decisions and show me when I
should serve and when I should step aside.

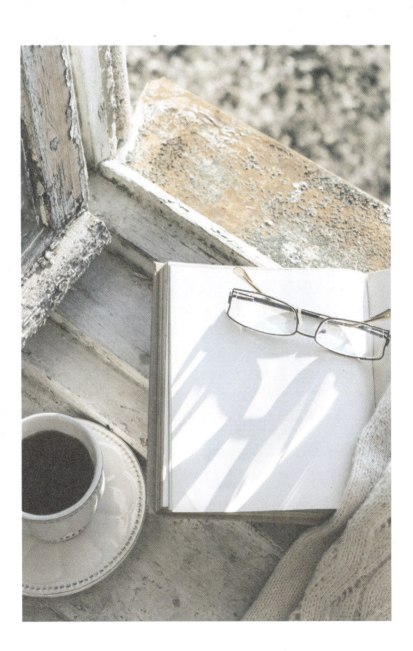

FEED YOUR BODY WITH REST

**God will meet all your needs according to
the riches of his glory in Christ Jesus.**
Philippians 4:19

When you look over the course of your day, are there times for rest? Are there moments you can catch your breath, sit down, and reflect? Or are you going and going until you drop into bed later than you'd hoped?

Dear friend, you need to rest every day. It might seem productive to rush around nonstop, but your body, mind, and soul were not created to function that way. Daily rest is needed, just like daily bread. If you skip eating, your body ends up depleted. In the same way, skipping rest leaves your body weak, weary, and, eventually, overwhelmed.

Incorporate rest into your daily routine. Follow the example of Jesus, who made an effort to rest even when thousands of people were looking to Him to be fed. Yes, He fed them with loaves and fishes, but then He also fed Himself with solitude, prayer, and rest (Matthew 14:23).

Jesus, help me follow Your example of taking time to rest.

OPPORTUNITY TO REST

Guide me in your truth and teach me, for you are God my Savior, and my hope is in you all day long.
Psalm 25:5

Pause for a moment. Feel your lungs fill as you breathe deeply. Roll your shoulders back and let them relax. Revel in the stillness. You might not have many moments like this in a day—moments to reflect in the silence and to sit without feeling guilty. Relish them.

Though these moments may be few and far between, they will happen throughout the day—while you're sitting in the school pickup line, waiting for your oil to be changed, or parking the car after a long day of work. Seize those fleeting moments, the ones so small that they could easily be missed, and let yourself rest for just a few seconds.

Breathe in and out. Thank God for His presence. Ask Him for His help. Look to Him for guidance. Allow your heart and your mind to center on Him. And take this opportunity to rest.

Father, help me find small pockets of
time to rest throughout my day.

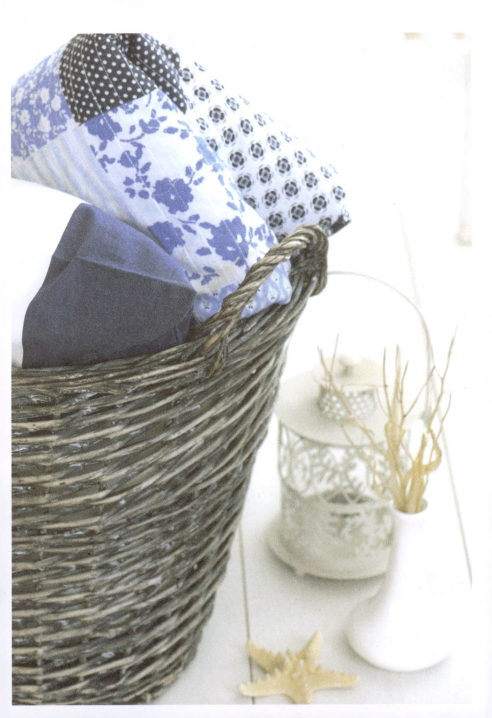

COUNT YOUR BLESSINGS

Now, our God, we give you thanks,
and praise your glorious name.
1 Chronicles 29:13

How often do you stop to count your blessings? It is so very easy to ignore what we have and focus on what we don't have. But a life of constant wanting leads to a life of constant striving. Be encouraged to find rest through thanksgiving today.

When you choose to focus on all that you *do* have, from the tiniest blessings to the biggest, your heart can't help but rejoice. A cool shower after an afternoon in the sun, a car that safely transports you to work, healthy children, food on the table—these are daily blessings.

Pause for a few minutes today and give thanks to the Lord, for He is good. All the good things in your life are His blessings to you—from the fragrant roses in your front yard to your closest confidant. He is a good God who loves to give good gifts to His children. Rest in thanksgiving today.

For all Your blessings, love, and mercy, I
give thanks to You, Most High God.

BE ON GUARD

**Above all else, guard your heart, for
everything you do flows from it.**
Proverbs 4:23

If you've ever watched a lifeguard on patrol, you've noticed that he or she scans the water constantly. Being a lifeguard requires diligence, focus, and discipline.

Just as a lifeguard guards a pool, you need to guard your schedule diligently. Say yes intentionally and say no gently but firmly. Refusing to let your schedule become overcrowded ensures that you have time for the people and things most important to you.

Guarding your schedule doesn't mean excluding people from your life or never helping when asked; rather, it allows you to be more thoughtful and prayerful in what you agree to take on. It helps you avoid burnout, and it allows you to create time for rest and rejuvenation. This is actually doing a favor not only to yourself but also to your family, friends, and community. Because the more rested you are, the less you're stressed and the more you're able to give of yourself to those you love.

Father, I offer up my day to You. Show
me what You would have me do.

PLAN A REST-FILLED WEEK

**And which of you by being anxious can
add a single hour to his span of life?**
Matthew 6:27 ESV

The days have a tendency to fly by, leaving you out of breath and out of energy, and you're not sure how to change your situation. Have you ever considered structuring your week so it's more conducive to rest?

Make a schedule at the beginning of the week that includes all your must-do items. As you list them, ask yourself if any of the items can be shared or altered. Can you figure out a carpool for your kids? Can you share meal preparation with a spouse or friend? Can you better use the alone time you do have—during your commute, early in the morning, or on your lunch break?

After seeing the structure of your week, you may be able to tweak it and allow yourself a time of rest every day. A week with downtime won't simply fall into your waiting arms; it takes discipline and planning, but it will be worth it.

""""""""""""

You, Lord, are a God of order. Help me bring
order and rest to my life this week.

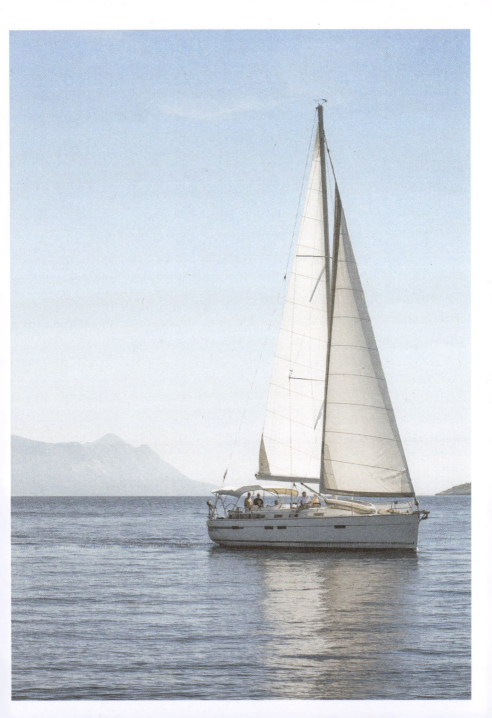

FINDING REST IN UNAVAILABILITY

The LORD longs to be gracious to you; therefore he will rise up to show you compassion.
Isaiah 30:18

*T*ired. Exhausted. Worn out. Overworked. Stressed. Too busy. If those words describe you, it may be time to be unavailable for a bit. You need to create margin and space in your life, and sometimes the only way to do that is by saying no.

You want to help others and be involved. You love feeling needed and productive. But there comes a time when you need to say, "No more."

Consider declaring yourself unavailable for a season. Do your work and do it well. Love your family and God and love them well. But put everything else by the wayside for a time. Being unavailable isn't a lifelong status, and it won't cause the world to spin off its axis. Instead, it will create space in your life for you to be refreshed, to pray more, and to love more deeply. Most importantly, putting the Lord first will bring the inner peace that your heart and soul need.

Lord, teach me when I should be available and when I should be unavailable.

THE PRESENT DAY

*Everyone was amazed and gave praise to
God. They were filled with awe and said,
"We have seen remarkable things today."*
Luke 5:26

How often do you think about the next hour, day, month, or year? How often have you thought, *I can't wait until . . . ?* Have you ever found yourself wishing that today would hurry up and be over so that you can get on with your real life? It's understandable, but try to remember that this present day is God's gift to you. Open it up; enjoy it fully.

In this present moment, God gives you breath. He keeps your heart beating. He woke you up this morning, and He reveals Himself to you all throughout the day—through the kindness of a stranger, the colorful autumn leaves, the rich orange hue of pumpkins at the market. Don't be so focused on the future that you miss the present; it is filled with God's blessings and gifts. There is much to be enjoyed in this day. Look for it, then revel in the joy of this present moment.

Jesus, when I'm wishing time would pass by,
remind me that today is a gift from You.

LORD, HELP ME MAKE TIME TO REST...

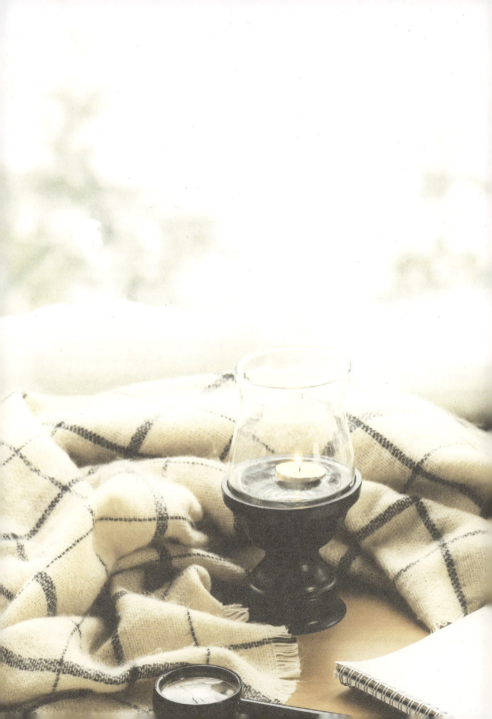

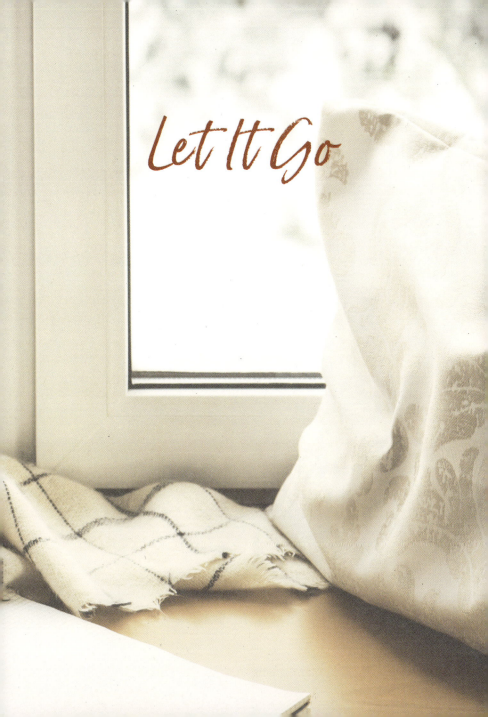

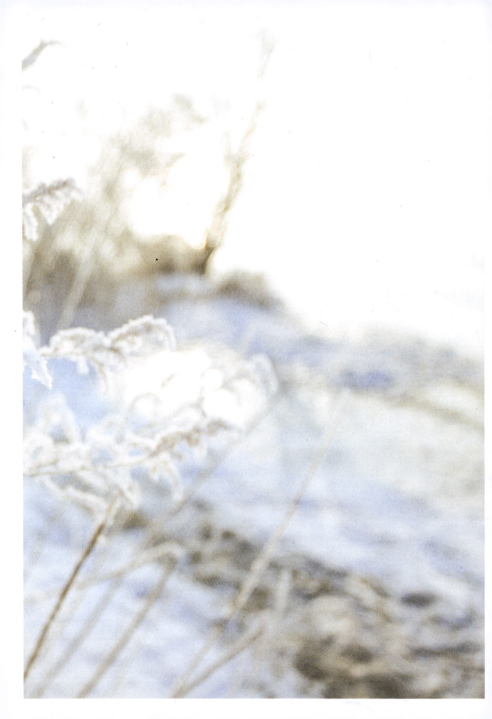

EASE YOUR EXPECTATIONS

Since we are surrounded by such a great cloud of witnesses, let us throw off everything that hinders and the sin that so easily entangles. And let us run with perseverance the race marked out for us.
Hebrews 12:1

You wanted to finish that big project at work, vacuum the house, take the car to the shop, check in with your dad, cook dinner, and get ahead on your Bible study. But none of those things happened, and you're left feeling really discouraged. We've all had those sorts of days.

You may need to adjust your expectations. Sometimes they're simply too high, and you run the risk of getting stuck in a vicious cycle of unmet expectations and disappointment. It's okay, at times, to throw your hands up and say, "I'll try again tomorrow."

Is it time to ease up on your expectations a little? Would it really be disastrous if you didn't finish everything today? God promises to always take care of you—and that promise doesn't end if your to-do list isn't finished. Let go of your expectations and, instead, ask God to help you look at your day through the lens of His expectations.

God, help me adjust my expectations and live according to Your plans, not my own.

IF YOU STEP AWAY . . .

As God's chosen people, holy and dearly loved, clothe yourselves with compassion, kindness, humility, gentleness and patience.
Colossians 3:12

If I'm not there, everything will fall apart. Many people feel this way about their responsibilities, whether they're a stay-at-home mom, an executive assistant, the president of a nonprofit, or a committed volunteer at the mission.

It's true—things might get a little chaotic if you aren't there. You might come back to more work, a frazzled spouse, or a little disarray. But you might not. And either way, life will go on—even without you there to guide, lead, prod, and pick up the slack.

If you are feeling stressed to the max because you believe you're indispensable, you might want to reevaluate the situation. Give someone else a chance to step up, practice responsibility, and increase their confidence, even as you allow yourself some much-needed rest. Take a step back and let things go for a day, or even just a few hours. Life will go on, and you'll come back feeling more equipped, capable, and energetic.

Lord, help me remember that the world won't
fall apart if I take time away to rest.

LET GO OF FEAR OF FAILURE

Restore our fortunes, LORD, like streams in the Negev.
Psalm 126:4

N o one likes to fail—but at some point in our lives, we all do. Maybe you've already snapped at your children three times today, or you completely forgot to prep for that important meeting. Perhaps you shared someone's secret, did poorly on a test, or forgot your mom's birthday.

Sometimes we're so afraid of failing that we try to be in control of every last detail. We believe complete control is the key to avoiding failure. But this is an illusion because we can never truly be completely in control.

The fact is, you will fail. You will mess up and make mistakes. When you do, apologize, forgive yourself, and move on. Don't battle for control; instead, let the Lord guide your steps. Talk with Him throughout the day. And when you fail, watch His grace step in and wash your mistakes away. Don't let fear of failing reign over your life.

I mess up every day, Father. Cover me with Your grace and remind me that You are in control.

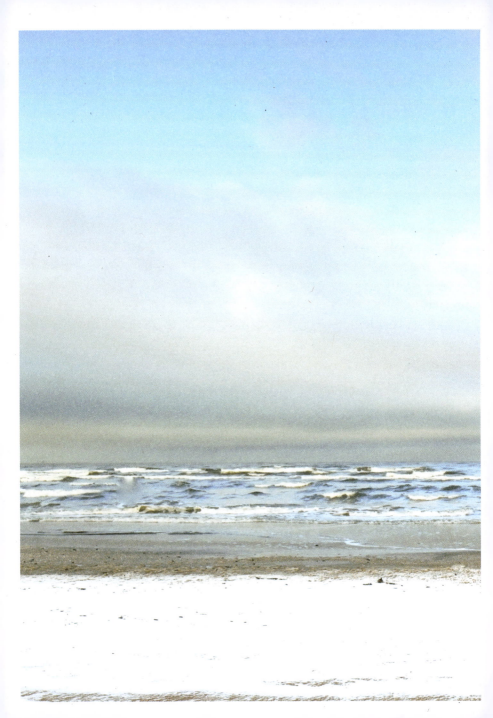

LET GO OF ANXIETY

**When anxiety was great within me,
your consolation brought me joy.**
Psalm 94:19

Anxiety is real. It is all-consuming and paralyzing; it can make you feel out of control, isolated, and fearful. Maybe you experience it on a daily basis, or perhaps you only have anxiety when you're flying in an airplane or riding in a taxi. Every person has varying degrees of anxiety in life, but the truth is simple: Anxiety can overtake you.

If you are feeling anxious today, there is hope. You can find relief, and you can overcome it. There will be a day when your heart won't race uncontrollably. There will be a time when you won't feel overwhelmed.

Start by asking God for help. Then seek out a family member, friend, or counselor. Fill your mind with scriptures about God's peace. And find hope knowing that your anxiety will not last forever. You will find rest.

Father, when anxiety threatens to consume me, lead
me to Your refuge and calm my troubled heart.

LET GO OF TROUBLES

Why, my soul, are you downcast? Why so
disturbed within me? Put your hope in God, for
I will yet praise him, my Savior and my God.
Psalm 42:5

In John 16:33, Jesus told His followers, "I have told you these things, so that in me you may have peace. In this world you will have trouble. But take heart! I have overcome the world." If you're in a time of trouble, do not be dismayed and do not be discouraged; Jesus is not surprised by it.

If your heart is downcast and your burden feels heavy, Jesus wants you to do something radical: He wants you to give your burden to Him. He wants to take it from you so that you are no longer beaten down or afraid. What a gift! What a Savior!

Jesus wants you to have rest during the joyful times of your life, but He also wants to give you peace when you're walking through the storms. In Christ alone your hope is found. Fall into His waiting arms! He can—and will—give rest to your soul.

O Father, sometimes the storms overwhelm me.
Thank You for the refuge of Your strong arms.

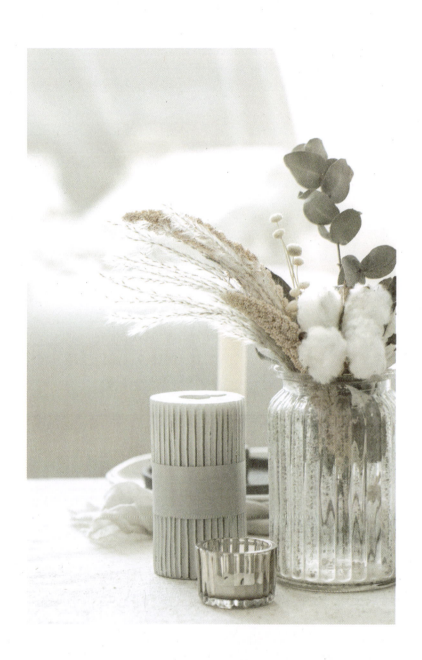

THE DEPTHS OF DESPAIR

**You gave abundant showers, O God; you
refreshed your weary inheritance.**
Psalm 68:9

Is your heart downcast? Is it full of worry and trouble? This world has so much heartache. Our families carry wounds, friends let us down, and loved ones pass away . . . Sometimes life seems too hard to handle. We live in a broken world. And we live among broken people.

You're doing your best in the fight against despair, but your prayers feel heavy. The weight of the struggle is dragging you down, and you're not sure if you have enough strength to get back up. You're tired and discouraged.

Take heart, for the Lord will rescue you. You can let that burden slide off your back; He promises to carry your heartache, your shame, and your sorrows. In the middle of this storm, remember that God promises to never leave or forsake you—and He means it. Find peace, dear one, as you rest in Christ alone.

Lord, I'm no match for life's trials. Please give me
rest, and comfort me with Your presence.

THE HARM OF COMPLAINING

Don't grumble against one another,
brothers and sisters, or you will be judged.
The Judge is standing at the door!
James 5:9

Sometimes complaining feels good, doesn't it? At least for a few minutes. But then you usually end up feeling even more frustrated, jaded, or angry than before. Complaining doesn't help you forget or move on; it solidifies your feelings of being wronged. And those feelings can take root deep inside you, hardening your heart.

Where there is complaining, there is no peace. Peace comes from a contented heart, from understanding that life isn't fair, and from choosing to embrace what life has to offer you. Peace is a restful state. Complaining, on the other hand, brings only weariness.

The next time you find yourself complaining, note how your body reacts. You may feel your blood pressure rise, your shoulders tighten, and your hands curl into fists. This isn't healthy or restful. Let go of your complaints, turn them over to God in prayer, and let Him replace them with peace and contentment . . . and rest.

Lord, please take this complaining spirit of mine
and replace it with peaceful trust in You.

WHATEVER IS TRUE

*Whatever is true, whatever is noble, whatever
is right, whatever is pure, whatever is lovely,
whatever is admirable—if anything is excellent
or praiseworthy—think about such things.*
Philippians 4:8

Anger. Jealousy. Self-contempt. Annoyance. How often do you think negatively? If you're stuck in a traffic jam, is your mind full of frustration toward other drivers? When your spouse disagrees with a decision you made, do you let bitterness overtake you? Do you often find yourself thinking more negatively than positively throughout the day? If so, then perhaps it's time to change the way you think.

It's easy—all too easy—to wallow in self-pity or to fixate on your own anger or someone else's issues. But in doing so, you rob yourself of the joy found in all that is true, noble, right, pure, lovely, admirable, excellent, and praiseworthy. If your mind is a swirling realm of destructive thoughts, there's no room for anything else.

Today, focus instead on what is true—that you are blessed by a God who loves you. Give your mind and body a break from negativity, and rest in the goodness of God.

*Father, guide my thoughts. Teach me to
focus on whatever is pure and true.*

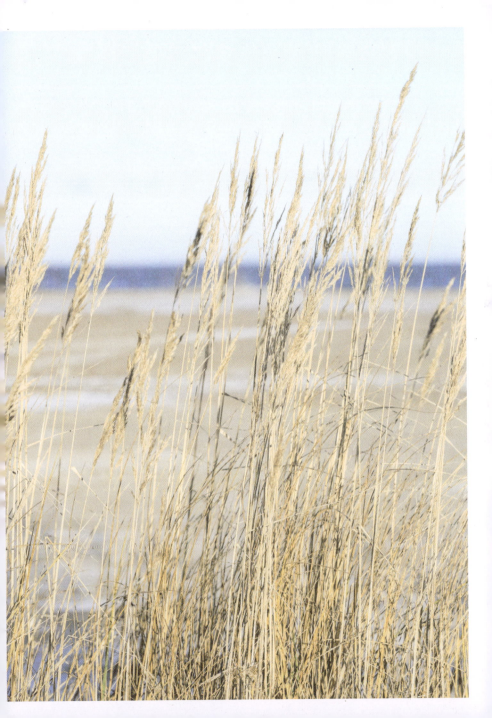

FREEDOM IN JESUS

Cast your cares on the LORD and he will sustain you; he will never let the righteous be shaken.
Psalm 55:22

What is weighing heavily on your heart today, friend? Do you feel especially anxious about something? Do you feel discouraged or frustrated about a particular situation? The Lord desires to give you rest from those burdens. He wants to free you from any anxiety or worry, and He wants to bless you with His peace, joy, and hope.

Whatever your worry—about yourself or a loved one, about health or money, about spiritual concerns—the Lord knows and cares. He lovingly tells us to bring Him those burdens and worries. He will take them on. Instead of feeling buried under the weight of anxiety, you can experience the freedom of hope.

Turn to Jesus. He knows you are worried and tired, and He longs for you to come to Him so that He can give you rest.

''''''''''''''''''''''''''''

Lord Jesus, I bring my worries to You,
and I trust You to take control.

BREATHING IN GOD'S PEACE

**Blessed are the peacemakers, for they
will be called children of God.**
Matthew 5:9

Have you ever noticed a physical reaction when you're worried? For many, a pounding heart, sweating, shaking, shortness of breath, difficulty swallowing, nausea, or dizziness may take hold of the body. It may not be obvious at first, but as your worries increase, the physical symptoms become stronger.

Have you felt any of those symptoms this week? Do you feel surprised by how well those words describe you? Beloved, this life has many worries, but our God is bigger and stronger than them all.

Take a deep breath. As you breathe in, remind yourself of God's promises and faithfulness. As you breathe out, imagine all your worries flowing out of your body—because where the Spirit of the Lord is, there is freedom and no place for worry. Continue this deep breathing until your body relaxes and the Lord calms you. God is bigger than any trouble or worry; ask Him to fill you with His Spirit of peace.

*I'm full of worry, but I know You're able to
take this from me. Come quickly, Lord.*

LORD, HELP ME LET GO ...

_____

_____

_____

_____

_____

_____

_____

_____

_____

_____

_____

_____

_____

_____

_____

_____

_____

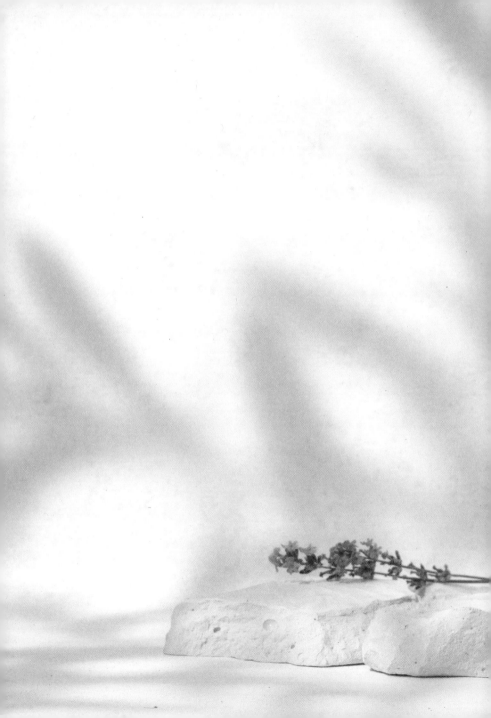

Rest Your Body

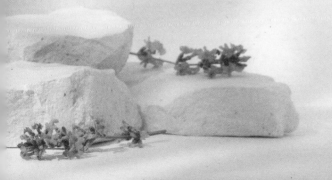

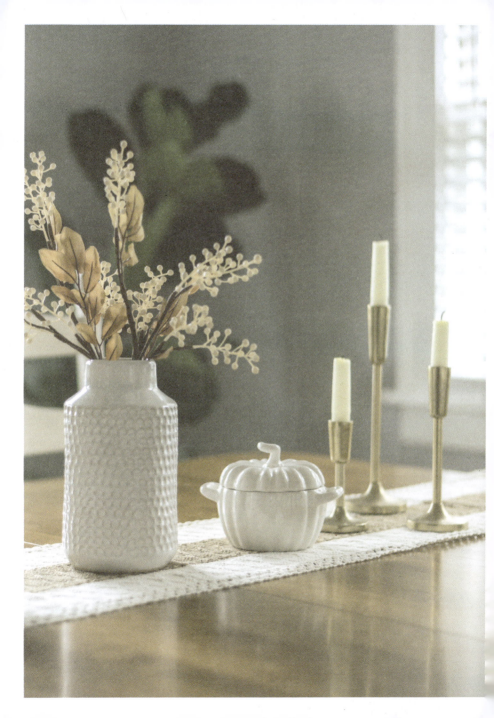

RESISTING STRESS

**Say to those who have an anxious
heart, "Be strong; fear not!"**
Isaiah 35:4 ESV

How often do you hear someone say, "I'm stressed"? Stress is interwoven in our modern lives. Yet the havoc it plays on our bodies is frightening. Heart disease, depression, digestive issues, autoimmune disorders, memory problems, and nervous habits are all effects of stress.

How can you combat stress in your life? It will take some effort. Try engaging your body in a physical activity like stretching. See a counselor, clear your calendar, get sufficient rest, and immerse yourself in prayer. Less busyness, more deep breathing, and fewer burdens will all lead to a life less marked by stress.

But first and always, when anxiety and stress threaten to overwhelm you, turn to the One who loves you best. Sit in the presence of the Most High God, and let Him lift away the tension in your body as you pray to Him. He can and will help you resist stress—and find rest.

I praise You, my King and my Maker, for You
know and provide exactly what I need.

INHALE, EXHALE, AND RELEASE

My heart is not proud, LORD, my eyes are not haughty; I do not concern myself with great matters or things too wonderful for me. But I have calmed and quieted myself.
Psalm 131:1–2

Did you know that when you're worried or stressed, you breathe differently? Your breaths become quick and shallow instead of even and deep, and you engage your shoulders instead of your diaphragm. Your jaw clenches and tightens.

You probably don't have time for a massage or the spa, but you want to feel better. You want your body and mind to feel at rest. That's where inhaling, exhaling, and releasing come in.

If your breathing is shallow, take several deep breaths in a row. Let your breath expand your lungs and move your diaphragm. As you exhale, do so slowly and in a controlled manner. If your jaw is tense, move it back and forth and do some stretches with it; you may feel a little silly, but you will also feel better. Throughout the day, do this breathing and jaw check. If you feel tension, then inhale, exhale, release . . . and rest in your breathing.

Father, remind me to inhale, exhale, and release whenever I feel anxious.

GO OUTSIDE

Since the creation of the world God's invisible
qualities—his eternal power and divine nature—
have been clearly seen, being understood from what
has been made, so that people are without excuse.
Romans 1:20

Many studies have shown that being outdoors is not only good for your physical well-being, it's also good for your mental and social well-being. Nature helps increase attention span, creativity, problem-solving skills, and self-esteem. It can reduce stress, increase conflict-resolution skills, strengthen immunity, raise test scores, and ease depression.

With all those benefits, why not go outside? The great outdoors is a great place to unwind and rest. Whether you take a long bike ride, walk along a hiking trail, jog around your neighborhood, or simply sit by the lake, you'll find great benefits in intentionally being outdoors.

God's creation is beautiful, restorative, inspiring, and soothing. If you're feeling stressed or simply in need of a break from everyday life, open the door and step outside. Relax in the wonders of being in the open air.

When I look at the work of Your hands,
Lord, my heart is full of wonder.

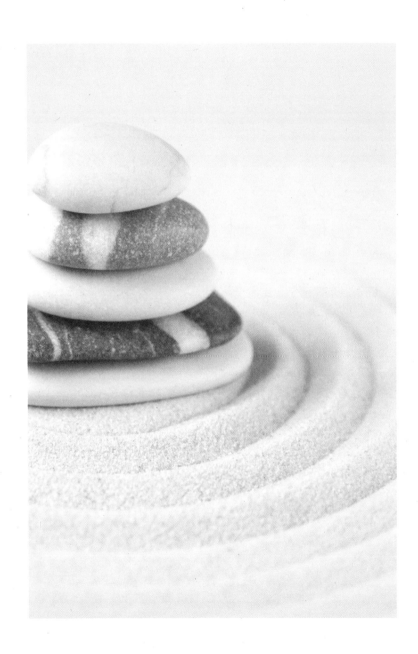

LISTEN TO YOUR BODY

*Praise the L*ORD*, my soul, and forget not all his
benefits—who forgives all your sins and heals all
your diseases, who redeems your life from the
pit and crowns you with love and compassion.*
Psalm 103:2–4

It's usually easy to tell when your body is getting sick. You feel aches and pains, and you might even begin to feel feverish. Perhaps you wake up with a sore throat, or you simply can't go another minute without a nap. When sickness is coming, your body gives you warning signs.

In the same way, when exhaustion is coming, your body will let you know. You may feel constantly fatigued, depressed, or discouraged. You may want to throw your alarm clock across the room when it wakes you in the morning. Listen to your body; it's time to start slowing down and allow yourself to rest.

Let yourself sleep for an extra hour. Ask for help on that overwhelming work project. Tell your spouse you need more help around the house or with the kids. Say no to more obligations. If your body is telling you to rest, listen—and then rest.

Lord, my body feels so weary. Bless me with rest today.

HEALING ON THE INSIDE

The LORD is good, a refuge in times of trouble.
He cares for those who trust in him.
Nahum 1:7

R ecovering from illness or injury takes time. And though the progress may not always be readily apparent, slowly and surely, the body does heal. After a while, the glow of health and strength returns.

The same can be said of a person in need of physical and spiritual rest. If you have been worn down by the demands of this life, remember that recovering from deep exhaustion takes time. And though the progress may not always be readily apparent, slowly and surely, your body and your spirit will heal.

As you lean on the Lord, rest, and recharge, you'll find your inner strength returning. Your shoulders slowly relax. Your eyes begin to shine. You laugh more easily. Don't be discouraged if the process takes more time than you'd hoped. The Lord is working in you to heal you, to give you rest, and to fill you with His peace that passes all understanding.

Father God, restore my body and my
soul to a place of restful peace.

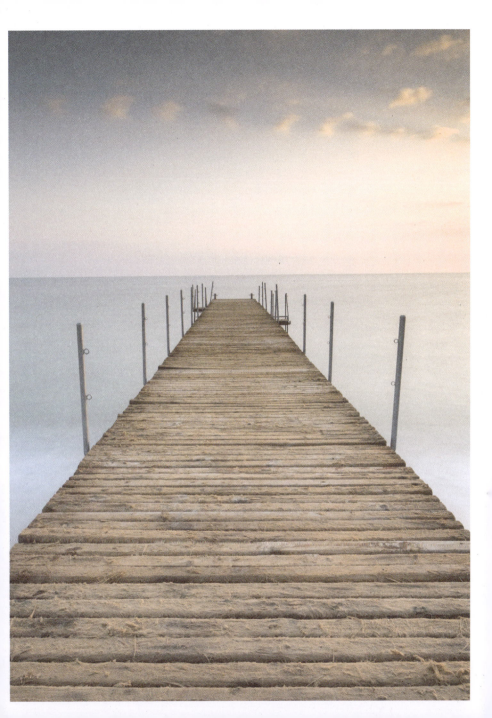

WHEN YOUR BODY SAYS NO

I praise you because I am fearfully and
wonderfully made; your works are
wonderful, I know that full well.
Psalm 139:14

God created each of us to be unique and wonderful. Our bodies are masterpieces, and they're designed to tell us when we're hungry, happy, sad, anxious, sick, or excited. They also tell us when we're tired.

When we are weary and exhausted, it shows physically. Dark circles appear under our eyes, our eyes sting with strain, our limbs feel sluggish, and our hearts sink when the alarm clock blares. Sound familiar?

When your body is telling you it's overwhelmed, what do you do? Do you try to push through and keep going until you reach your breaking point? Maybe you ignore the symptoms until you get physically ill. We live in a culture that glorifies busyness, but at some point, you really need to rest. Honor your body when it signals its tiredness. You are fearfully and wonderfully made. Respect your body and give yourself the rest you deserve.

You created our bodies so intricately, Father.
Help me honor Your creation with rest.

CARING FOR YOURSELF

I pray that from his glorious, unlimited
resources he will empower you with
inner strength through his Spirit.
Ephesians 3:16 NLT

Imagine yourself with a sweet child. But instead of treating that child with love and gentleness, you place high demands on her. You wake her after only a few hours of sleep, you make her scrub the floors without breakfast, and you allow her to eat only as you're rushing out the door. After school, you hand her an impossible to-do list—and when dinnertime comes and she hasn't completed it, you yell. You keep her up way past her bedtime and make her feel ashamed when she falls asleep on the couch. Who would treat a child that way?

But . . . is that the way you treat yourself?

Self-care is essential for living a healthy life, but it is so easy to neglect. Treat yourself like a child today: Relax your expectations, be kind to yourself, and rest when you get overwhelmed. Care for yourself.

Lord, help me tend to my own physical, spiritual,
and emotional needs as a parent tends to a child.

DON'T FORGET TO EAT

He made him ride on the heights of the land
and fed him with the fruit of the fields.
He nourished him with honey from the
rock, and with oil from the flinty crag.
Deuteronomy 32:13

R est for your soul is crucial, but rest and care for your body are important too. Did you know that Jesus made sure His disciples took time to rest and eat?

Mark 6:31 says, "Because so many people were coming and going that they did not even have a chance to eat, [Jesus] said to them, 'Come with me by yourselves to a quiet place and get some rest.'"

Jesus knew His disciples hadn't had a chance to eat, but instead of asking them to push through their hunger because their work was too important, He told them to leave the crowds and get some dinner.

Does this encourage you today? Jesus Himself told His disciples to pause in their ministering, to seek out a quiet place, to rest, and to nourish their bodies. How encouraging! The Lord wants to take care of you spiritually and physically too. Find time to sit in a quiet place, rest, and eat something healthy today.

Lord, remind me to rest and eat, just as You
did for the disciples so many years ago.

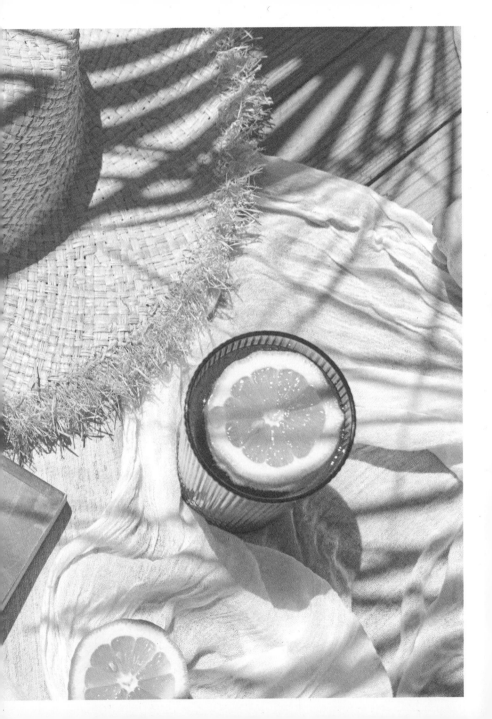

DON'T WAIT UNTIL IT'S TOO LATE

You will lie down, with no one to make you afraid.
Job 11:19

The physical effects of not getting enough sleep include impaired memory, increased blood pressure, increased risk of heart troubles, a weakened immune system, greater susceptibility to illness, weight gain, and type 2 diabetes—and that's just the tip of the iceberg!

That list is scary, but it's also accurate. When we push ourselves to the max, relying on coffee and carbs to get us through the day, we aren't doing ourselves any favors. And too often we wait until it's too late to rest. By then, our family is frustrated, our work is suffering, and our body is breaking down.

Don't wait until it's too late to rest. Be sure to get adequate sleep, ask friends to keep you accountable, and talk to the Lord about your worries. If you feel as if you simply can't rest, look to the One who watches over you. Ask Him to quiet your soul and lead you to rest.

Lord, I praise You because I am fearfully and wonderfully made. Help me take care of me.

SEEK PHYSICAL REST

*Even youths grow tired and weary, and young
men stumble and fall; but those who hope
in the LORD will renew their strength.*
Isaiah 40:30–31

How are you feeling physically? Does your body feel worn out? Is fatigue your constant companion? Do you collapse into bed at the end of the day? You need rest, dear friend, and you need it now.

Listen to your body. Rest is not a sign of weakness; in fact, recognizing and acting on the need for physical rest is one of the best things you can do for your body. If you're utterly exhausted, it's time to slow down.

Find solitude in a quiet place every day. It might be on your couch in the early morning hours, or it may come late at night, after everyone else is in bed. Instead of adding another event to the calendar, add rest. It may mean saying no—even to some good things—but you'll be saying yes to rest. Be still in the quiet, let the day's worries roll off your shoulders, and allow your body and mind to rest.

Father, help me remember to take advantage
of these quiet times with You.

LORD, HELP ME REST MY BODY ...

_____

_____

_____

_____

_____

_____

_____

_____

_____

_____

_____

_____

_____

_____

_____

_____

_____

_____

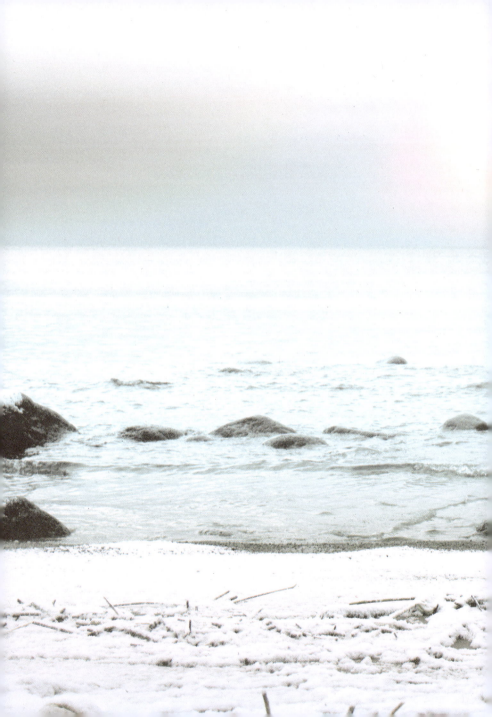

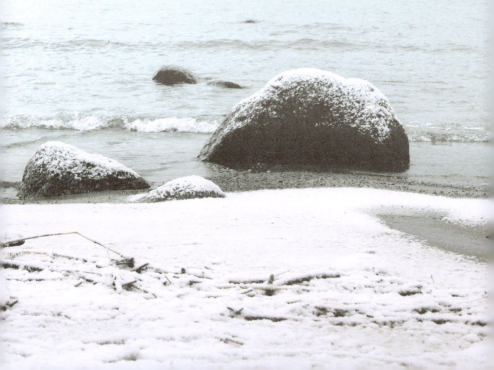

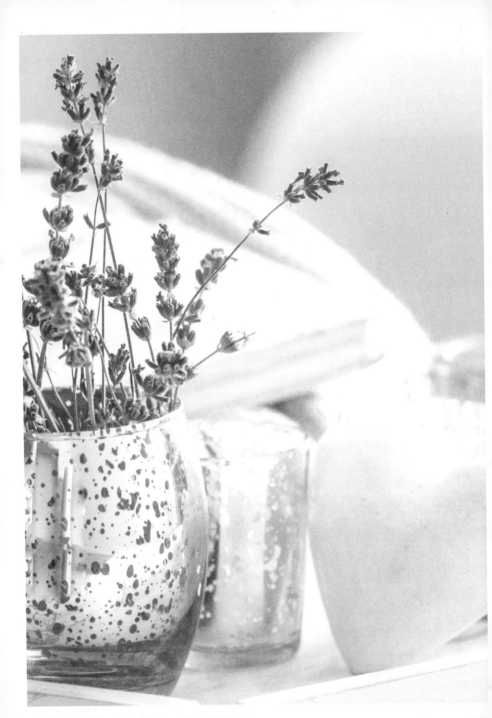

GIVE WORRY TO THE LORD

**Seek his kingdom, and these things
will be given to you as well.**
Luke 12:31

When you're worried, the stress of those cares can easily take over your life. Your thoughts drift in conversation, your heart beats faster, and you feel anxious and overwhelmed.

What are you anxious about today? Is it money? Fitting in with others? Finding a spouse? Difficulties with your job? Current events on the news?

Rest assured, the Lord knows your worries and anxieties. He hears you when you're afraid and hurting, and He wants to take this burden you're carrying. Cry out to Him today. Be specific. Ask Him to free you from this anxiety. His response may not be instant—you might not even feel very different at first—but you can be sure that the Lord is moving heaven and earth to rescue you. All you need to do is call out to Him. Give Jesus your worry today. It's never too much for Him to handle, and He will give you peace.

Please help me release my worries to You,
Lord. Remind me that You're in control.

THE BIG PICTURE

Consider how the wild flowers grow. They do not labor or spin. Yet I tell you, not even Solomon in all his splendor was dressed like one of these.
Luke 12:27

Have you ever helped with a big event? Maybe you planned the whole thing, or you were one of many tasked with helping execute the plan. Big events require so many details and decisions. It can be easy to get caught up in the most minute aspects and lose sight of the reason behind it all: the charity behind the golf tournament, the person honored by the party, the couple in love versus the show of the wedding.

The same thing can happen in life. There are so many details, both big and small, that can consume our lives: bills, retirement planning, vacations, kids and college, appointments, and relationships. All the details of life can certainly seem overwhelming, but in the grand scheme of things, life is about glorifying God and living for Him.

Instead of stressing over all the details of life, why not simply look at the big picture: God. Find relief in trusting Him with the details.

Lord God, remind me that life is less about
all the details and more about You.

PERFECT FOCUS

**Turn my eyes from looking at worthless
things; and give me life in your ways.**
Psalm 119:37 ESV

Does your future look blurry? Are you uncertain of the direction your life is (or should be) taking? We all deal with that at one time or another. But take comfort. God is an expert at bringing blurry futures into perfect focus. He usually does it one step at a time, so it can be scary. But you can trust His vision for your life.

In those times when your future seems blurry and uncertain, turn to God for direction. He promises that He'll never forsake those who seek Him. He will never leave you lost and wandering. Rest in the guidance He will give you, trusting Him day by day, moment by moment, step by step.

If you are a follower of Christ, the Lord is with you always. He won't let you down, and He'll never forget your needs. Rest in knowing that the Lord will bring perfect focus to your life when you seek Him.

———————————

When my future looks blurry, I trust that
You're in control and guiding my life, Lord.

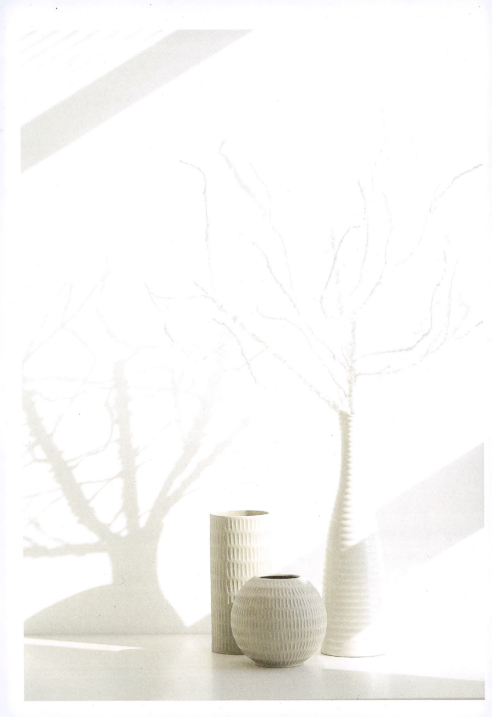

GOD, THE GIVER OF REST

**The Lord is my helper; I will not be afraid.
What can mere mortals do to me?**
Hebrews 13:6

When you hold tightly to your own plans, hopes, and dreams, you exhaust yourself. Why? Because you're pursuing your path according to your own strength, and your own strength is finite. It is limited. You are only human—you are not invincible—and your resources, though they may seem vast at times, are so very small when compared to the Lord's.

Trust in the Lord. His plans are bigger, better, and more beautiful than you could ever imagine. He doesn't want you to walk around worried and burdened and overwhelmed; instead, He wants you to rest in Him. Let God call the shots, make the plan, and work all things out for your good. Follow Him in complete trust. God alone is the Giver of gifts and the Giver of rest.

Lord, doing things my own way is exhausting.
Teach me to trust You and Your plans.

TRUSTING WITH ANTICIPATION

Peace I leave with you; my peace I give you. I do not give to you as the world gives. Do not let your hearts be troubled and do not be afraid.
John 14:27

*W*hen will it happen? How will this end? Is it almost over? When we're stuck in a time of waiting, we ask these questions over and over again. We want to know how much longer we'll be in this place and how our story will unfold. Surely the waiting would be easier if we knew the basic blueprint. Then we'd know how to prepare ourselves— we'd know if we need to buck up and push through, steel ourselves for disappointment, walk away, or celebrate. But the Lord knows that even the basic blueprint would overwhelm us. So He calls us to trust.

God wants you to trust Him wholeheartedly and without reservation. How can you do that? By believing that He is a good and gracious God, that He is perfect and loving, and that you are His beloved child for whom He has only good plans. Trust in His goodness; rest in His plans.

Lord God, I surrender my plans and questions
and ask that You teach me to trust You.

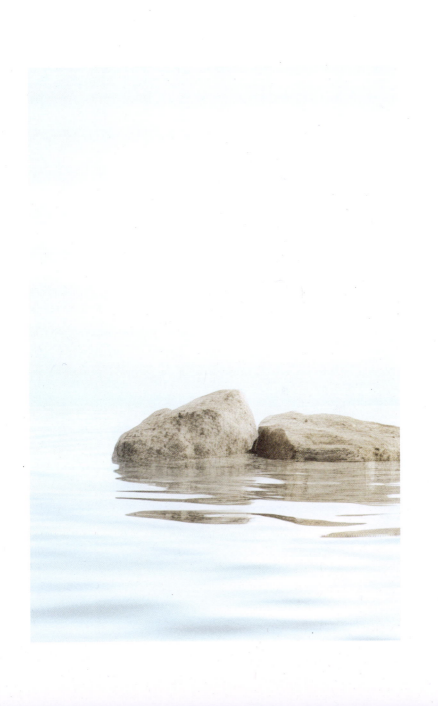

THE UNKNOWN FUTURE

**There is surely a future hope for you,
and your hope will not be cut off.**
Proverbs 23:18

It would be nice to know exactly what the future holds. That would take such a load of worry and fear off your shoulders, right? Or would it make you even more fearful?

Yes, there are surely exciting and wonderful things waiting for you in the future. But because we live in a sinful world, there will also be trials ahead. There will be scary and uncharted territory, pain, and confusion. Knowing all the difficult things you'll face might be more than your heart can handle right now.

God understands your hopes and concerns for the future, but He also knows you can't handle it all at once. God will faithfully provide everything you need to walk with Him each day. He just asks that you trust Him, one day at a time. No, you can't know the future. But you can know and trust the One who does.

*Father, You know my future and all its joys and
pain. I trust You to guide me through it.*

ARE WE THERE YET?

For the revelation awaits an appointed time; it speaks of the end and will not prove false. Though it linger, wait for it; it will certainly come and will not delay.
Habakkuk 2:3

A re we there yet?" Any parent knows that taking a trip with children means fielding this question at least a dozen times. And the answer often sounds like this: "No, we're still in the driveway," or "We've been in the car for ten minutes—we have ten more hours." The ridiculousness of the question makes us laugh, but the truth is we often ask God the same question.

When we're in a waiting period, we want to know when we'll arrive at our destination. "Is this suffering almost over, Lord?" "How much longer will this take?" "I've been waiting forever." Like impatient children, we don't understand that it often takes time to reach the good places in life.

So the next time you're tempted to ask the Lord, "Are we there yet?" remind yourself instead of His perfect timing. And if the answer is "Not yet," settle back and wait, knowing that He is the Master Driver.

I trust that You're working out a perfect plan, Jesus.
Give me the patience to endure the journey.

HE HOLDS THE FUTURE

We live by faith, not by sight.
2 Corinthians 5:7

The Maker of the stars and the heavens, the One who formed the trees and the mountains, the God who breathed life into man—He is the One who holds your future. He is creative. He is strong. He is almighty and all-powerful. And He loves and cares for you.

His plans may not always make sense to you, and the path you're on may feel foreign. Perhaps life has surprised you with all its joys and sorrows. But the Lord knows your every moment, every thought, and every desire; He rejoices in your joys and counts your every tear. And His faithfulness shines each evening in the majesty of the setting sun.

Child of God, your future is in good hands—the Lord's hands. Only He is able to turn night into morning, sorrow into dancing. Find rest in getting to know the God who holds your future. He is trustworthy. He is good. And He is able.

O Lord my God, I trust You to lead me and
guide me on this path home to You.

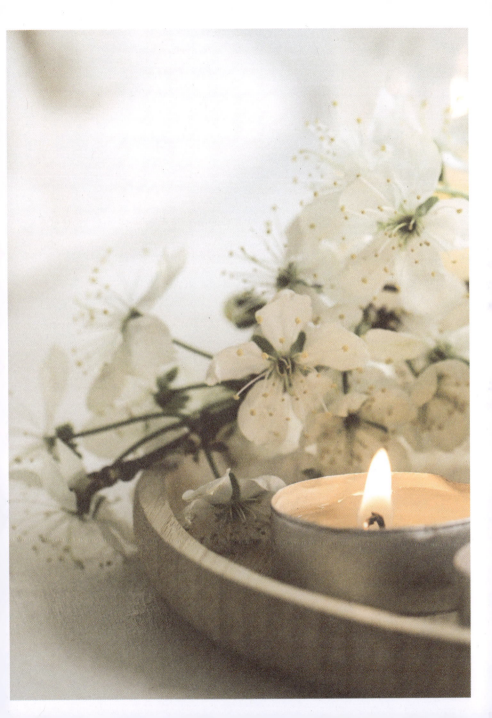

THE MONEY TREE

Where your treasure is, there your heart will be also.
Matthew 6:21

Wouldn't it be great if money really did grow on trees? Then every time you needed—or simply wanted—something, you could walk outside, grab some money, and head for the store. It would certainly make that Christmas shopping list easier to handle. Life, however, doesn't work that way, and that's probably a good thing. If we had all the money we ever wanted, we wouldn't know how to rely on the Lord.

So often it's the poorest people who have the deepest trust in God. Why? Because they've seen Him provide for them over and over again. When we feel as if we're providing for ourselves, we risk trusting in ourselves and in our own abilities instead of trusting in God, the ultimate Provider.

Instead of a money tree, the Lord has given you something far greater: Through Christ, you've been given the gift of a relationship with the One who created the trees. Rest in that truth and trust Him to supply all your needs.

*Lord, may I fully rest in Your provision
instead of trusting in my own abilities.*

H-E-L-P

The wisdom that comes from heaven is first of all pure; then peace-loving, considerate, submissive, full of mercy and good fruit, impartial and sincere.
James 3:17

*H*elp. It's a short word, but for many, it's so difficult to say. But asking for help isn't about helplessness. Asking for help is about **H**onesty, **E**nlisting others, the **L**ove of God, and **P**rayer.

Honesty means acknowledging that you are human and you can't do it all. You don't have infinite time, energy, brain space, or resources. So at times you need to enlist others, which means actively reaching out for help. It isn't shameful; it's a step toward living a more restful life. And it allows others the freedom to admit that they need help too.

You can also enlist God's help, trusting that He will provide it. Why? Because of His enormous love for you. How do you seek God's assistance? Through prayer. Open your mouth and heart, and spill out all your worries and struggles before the Lord.

Seek Him, seek H-E-L-P, and find rest.

―――――――――

Lord, give me the humility, honesty, and
courage to reach out for help.

LORD, HELP ME TRUST YOU . . .

_____

_____

_____

_____

_____

_____

_____

_____

_____

_____

_____

_____

_____

_____

_____

_____

_____

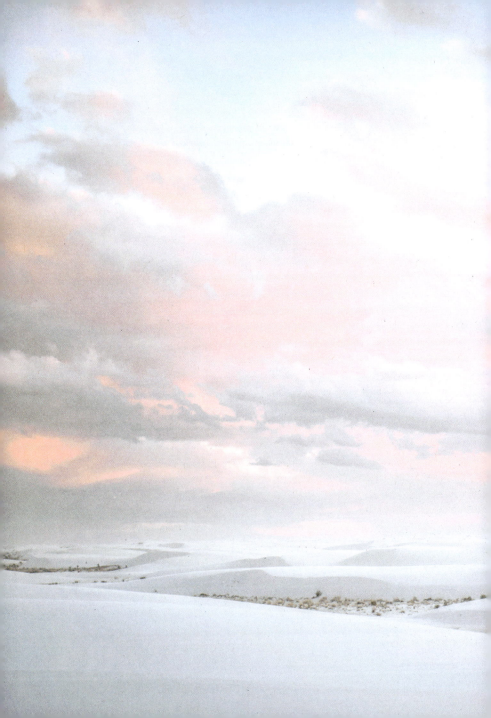

Do Not Worry or Fear

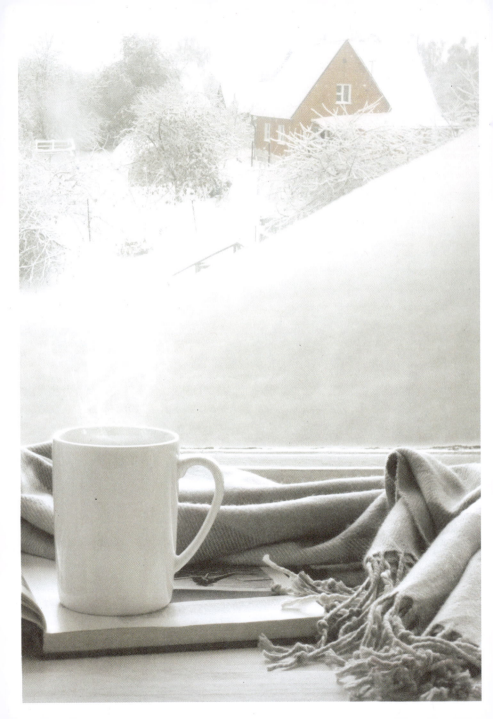

EVERY DAY HAS GOODNESS

Let us hold unswervingly to the hope we profess, for he who promised is faithful.
Hebrews 10:23

At the end of the day, do you feel defeated by the things you weren't able to accomplish? Even the best-laid plans can fail because life is unpredictable and messy. If you aren't able to finish everything you need or want to get done today, it can still be a good day. You do not need to feel defeated.

Think about all that you *were* able to do and experience today, from the smallest to the largest thing. Maybe you made the bed and put bread in the toaster. You got the children clothed and out to the bus on time. You made a casserole or mowed the lawn for someone who's sick. You encouraged a colleague. You laughed with your mom. You reassured a friend.

Every day has good in it because Christ is in every day. Don't allow disappointment to rule your thoughts. Celebrate the good you experience and thank God for blessing you with another day.

Thank You for being with me, Lord, through
both the highs and the lows of every day.

GOD'S BIG PROMISES

**Do not fear, for I am with you; do not be dismayed,
for I am your God. I will strengthen you and help
you; I will uphold you with my righteous right hand.**
Isaiah 41:10

God gives us big promises in the Bible: He promises never to leave or forsake us. He promises redemption and restoration to those who follow Him. And He promises that He has great plans and big dreams for us—greater than we could ever imagine. He declares that we are His masterpieces.

All of the Lord's promises are so good and so true, yet we live as though He's lying. We live frantically, striving and struggling to achieve our goals, prove ourselves, and attain approval. We say yes to too many things and no to too few for fear that others won't like us. Simply put, we aren't resting in God's promises.

The Lord tells us not to worry or be anxious; He'll provide for our every need. He tells us He delights in us, for we are His sons and daughters. How miraculous! How wonderful! Rest in the enduring, eternal, and perfect promises of God today.

*Teach me to trust Your promises; teach me
to delight in Your love for me, Father.*

TRUST GOD WITH YOUR FUTURE

Do not worry about tomorrow.
Matthew 6:34

G od knows the future—how long you will live, who you will love, every triumph you will celebrate, and every failure you will suffer. He is intricately involved in every single moment of your life, and He is working each of those moments together for His glory. Even so, the future can still be scary.

That's because, for us humans, the future is uncertain. No one knows when this life will end, if that loved one will survive the cancer, or if a child will make good choices. No one can predict the job market or the stock market, and no one knows when natural disasters or national tragedies will strike.

No, you can't know the future, but the One who calls you His beloved child does know. The One who calms your fears and wipes away your tears knows what you will need to face that future. Release your fears and find comfort in knowing that the One who holds the future in His hands also holds you.

Father, I am often afraid of the future. Remind me that You hold the future—and me—in Your hands.

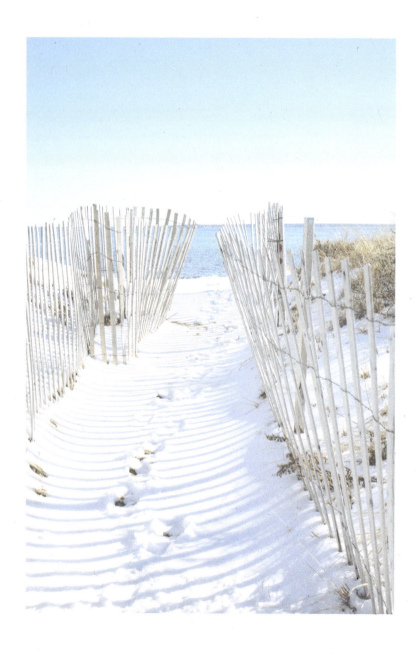

FAITH OVER FEAR

Trust in the LORD forever, for the LORD,
the LORD himself, is the Rock eternal.
Isaiah 26:4

Fear is invisible, but it is extremely powerful. Like a spider's web, it clings to everything it touches. It can be paralyzing, overwhelming, all-encompassing, and life-altering. Fear runs rampant in our world.

But as God's beloved children, we do not need to give way to fear. It doesn't have to be a part of our lives. Instead, we can rest in peaceful confidence, knowing that the almighty God of the universe takes care of us. He holds us in the palm of His hand—the same hand that filled the oceans and flung the stars into the farthest reaches of the heavens. He, the One who never grows weary, watches over us while we sleep and commands the sun to rise up to greet us each morning. The Lord our God is greater than all our fears.

Let go of your fears today. Lay them at the feet of God. Breathe in His promises of provision and exhale any doubt. The Lord is faithful to protect His children. Rest in His faithfulness to you.

I give my fears to You, Lord Jesus. Thank
You for Your promised relief and peace.

IN THE DARK OF NIGHT

**The sun will no more be your light by day, nor
will the brightness of the moon shine on you,
for the LORD will be your everlasting light.**
Isaiah 60:19

Have you ever found yourself in pitch-black darkness, unable to see where you're going? You strain your eyes, feel around with your hands, and tense your muscles while trying not to trip or stumble. You can't relax because you're not sure where you are.

But what if someone were guiding you by the hand, and you had a flashlight? Your experience would be totally different, wouldn't it? You'd be able to see the way ahead. It would be much less stressful.

Dear friend, the Lord is guiding you. His Word is a lamp for your feet, a light for your way. He knows exactly how to get you where you need to go, and He is the most trustworthy guide; He has an aerial view. You can have peace, knowing that the Creator of the universe is guiding you along in His perfect, redemptive plan. You can find rest, even in the darkness.

*Lord, teach me to trust Your leading instead
of fumbling around on my own.*

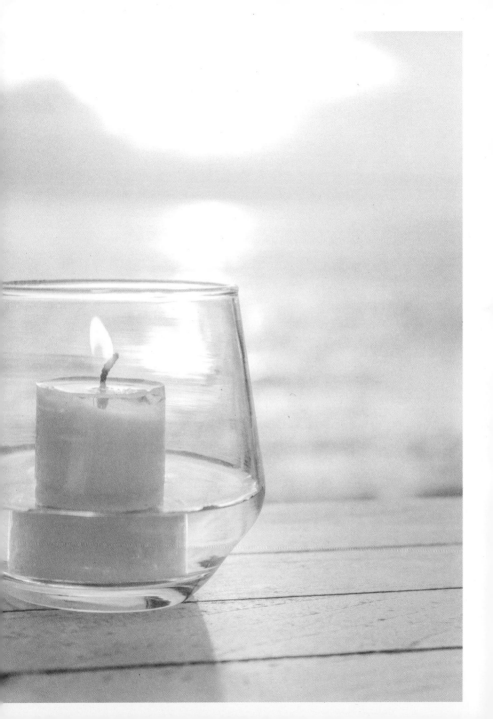

GOD IS BIGGER

We are hard pressed on every side, but not crushed;
perplexed, but not in despair; persecuted, but not
abandoned; struck down, but not destroyed.
2 Corinthians 4:8–9

Before Jesus left this earth, He said, "In this world you will have trouble. But take heart! I have overcome the world" (John 16:33). Jesus stated a fact: We will have trouble. Life will be hard. So if you're feeling as if life is just one battle after another, that doesn't surprise Jesus. He predicted it long ago, and it's still true for His followers today. But Jesus didn't leave us to wallow in that trouble; instead, He gave us hope.

We have hope because, through His death and resurrection, He has already overcome the world. We don't need to worry, fear, or despair. We know how the story will end—with Jesus' complete victory!

If you are weakening under a heavy load of troubles, take heart because the Lord is stronger. He is bigger. He is your Deliverer and Provider, and He can give you rest from despair.

Jesus, I cling to You and to Your words of
encouragement. Thank You for being my refuge.

YOU ARE NOT FORSAKEN

Those who know your name trust in you, for you,
LORD, have never forsaken those who seek you.
Psalm 9:10

In your darkest moments, you may feel forsaken by God. You might feel that your prayers are falling on deaf ears, or maybe you think God simply doesn't care about you anymore. Have you ever felt forsaken?

Dear friend, you are not forsaken—and you will never be forgotten. You may be in a dark valley, and it may look as if your prayers have not been answered, but even in the darkness, the Lord is by your side.

Cast away fear and unrest, raise your hands to your heavenly Father, and ask Him to make Himself known to you. He clearly says in His Word that He does not forsake those who seek Him; may you fully understand that truth. The Lord has not forgotten you; He is not ignoring you or turning a deaf ear to your cries. Rest in His arms. He is a loving, faithful, and always-present God. Hallelujah!

When I feel forgotten, may I remember Your promise
to never leave or forsake me, Father God.

TRUST IN GOD'S PROVISION

**Do not worry about your life, what you will eat;
or about your body, what you will wear. For life is
more than food, and the body more than clothes.**
Luke 12:22–23

E ven the rich worry about money. Businesses rise and fall every day; there could be a stock market crash or a sudden shift in consumer interest. Even if you have millions in the bank, money can still be a constant source of stress. And those who struggle to make ends meet have even more serious concerns about the money that buys their clothes, puts food on their table, and keeps a roof over their heads.

Money can be worrisome for the rich, the poor, and everyone in between. Would you like a rest from worrying about money? The Lord is willing and able to take away your burden. Whether you are worried about losing money, wondering how in the world to make money, or feeling anxious about your next meal, the Lord understands. And He says, "Do not worry." He knows what you need, and He promises to provide for you. Claim that promise today.

*Father, please take away my worry about
money. Replace it with trust in You.*

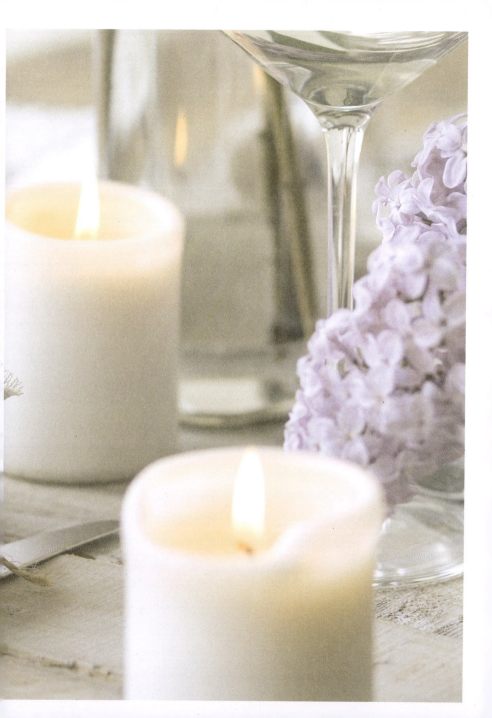

WHEN FINANCES LOOK BLEAK

Some trust in chariots and some in horses, but
we trust in the name of the LORD our God.
Psalm 20:7

You swipe your credit card to pay for groceries and inwardly wince. You put your tithe in the offering plate at church and pray the Lord will provide. You pick up all the odd jobs you can find, and you're an expert on coupons. Still, your finances look bleak.

If you're wrestling with money worries, hear these words: God knows your needs. He knows how much those car repairs will cost, how long you'll be unemployed, and when the next tuition payment is due. He's intimately involved in your life, and He cares deeply about you and your well-being.

Take a deep breath and feel the air rush through your lungs. The Lord—who formed your airways and the very oxygen molecules that fill them—knows everything you need, and He promises to provide. Cling to His promises today. When your finances look bleak, rest in the provision of the cross.

You promise to provide for me, Lord, and
I am choosing to trust Your words.

THE LORD GOES BEFORE YOU

It is the LORD who goes before you. He will be with you; he will not leave you or forsake you. Do not fear or be dismayed.
Deuteronomy 31:8 ESV

W hen you look ahead into the future days and weeks, you may feel overwhelmed. There are appointments, obligations, social events, and so many demands on your time. Your heart pounds as you wonder, *How will I get through this day, let alone the next week?*

When Moses was speaking to the fearful Israelites, he said in Deuteronomy 31:6, "Be strong and courageous. Do not fear or be in dread of them, for it is the LORD your God who goes with you. He will not leave you or forsake you" (ESV). Dear friend, those words are also for you.

And not only does the Lord promise to be with you, He also promises to go before you. He knows what you will be up against in the next hour, in the next week, in the next decade. And He goes before you to prepare the way. What a comfort!

Today, trust God to give you the wisdom and resources to meet this day's challenges. Rest in His promised provision.

Lord, thank You for going before me.
I will trust in You today.

LORD, HELP ME NOT TO WORRY OR FEAR...

_____

_____

_____

_____

_____

_____

_____

_____

_____

_____

_____

_____

_____

_____

_____

_____

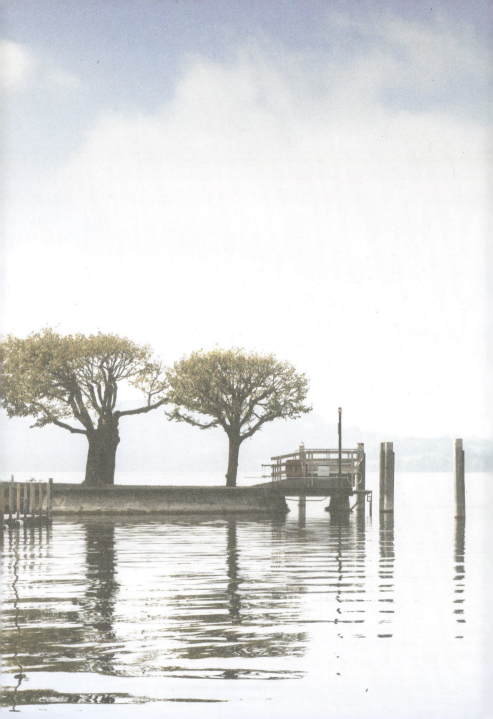

Find Contentment

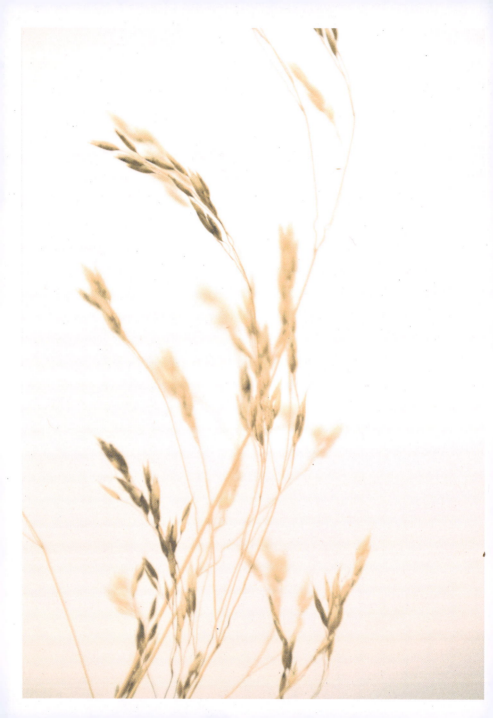

FIND JOY IN THE LORD

**You have been my hope, Sovereign LORD,
my confidence since my youth.**
Psalm 71:5

We look for joy and fulfillment in many places: a new house, our career, a relationship, a child, a hobby. While these things can certainly bring us happiness, they can't give us the deep, soul-stirring, everlasting joy and contentment we crave. Do you find yourself wanting more? Do you feel a yearning that you can't quite fill? That's your desire for God.

You can have the nicest clothes, biggest salary, most loving family, or largest social group, but without a deep satisfaction in the Lord, you'll feel empty. You won't feel joyful or at rest; you'll feel hollow. Does that resonate with you?

Ask the Lord to fill you with the joy that can only come from Him. Make spending time with Him a priority and converse with Him throughout your day. We all have a longing within us that can only be filled by God, and He's waiting to fill it. He's waiting to give you joy—and rest.

O Lord, fill this hole in my life with
Your presence and Your joy.

CREATURES OF DISCONTENT

**I was young and now I am old, yet I
have never seen the righteous forsaken
or their children begging bread.**
Psalm 37:25

If you find yourself struggling to be content, it's not surprising. We are bombarded with messages that we don't have enough. Advertisers tell us the happiest people have the newest car, latest phone, biggest wardrobe, and largest bank account. We are discontented creatures, and it all began with Adam and Eve.

When Satan appeared to Adam and Eve and said they could have even more—they could be *like God*—they wanted it. They saw the one thing they didn't have, they set their sights on it, and they sinned. Discontentment prompted the first sin, and sometimes we feel as if it cannot be overcome. But take courage: God can bring contentment to your heart.

Are you tired of striving for more? Find peace for your soul by turning to the Lord. When you feel discontentedness creeping in, ask God to show you true fulfillment in Him.

I think I know what I need, Lord, but You truly
know what I need. Show me Your fulfillment.

CHOOSE CONTENTMENT

**Do not work for food that spoils, but
for food that endures to eternal life,
which the Son of Man will give you.**
John 6:27

Socrates once said, "He who is not contented with what he has would not be contented with what he would like to have." So often we think that if we just had a new house, different job, new wardrobe, better-behaving kids, more money, or even a different spouse, we would be happier, we would be content. But would we?

Contentment is a choice; it doesn't magically happen. It doesn't automatically come with a new job or a new pair of jeans. If you want to be released from discontent, you must choose to be content.

Contentment begins with gratitude. If you focus on what you *don't* have, you immediately become less grateful for all you do have. The Lord knows it's a struggle, and He wants to untangle you from the trap of discontentment. Call on Him today. Ask Him to give you freedom, contentment, and peace.

O Father, I struggle with being content. Please
free me from the trap of discontentment.

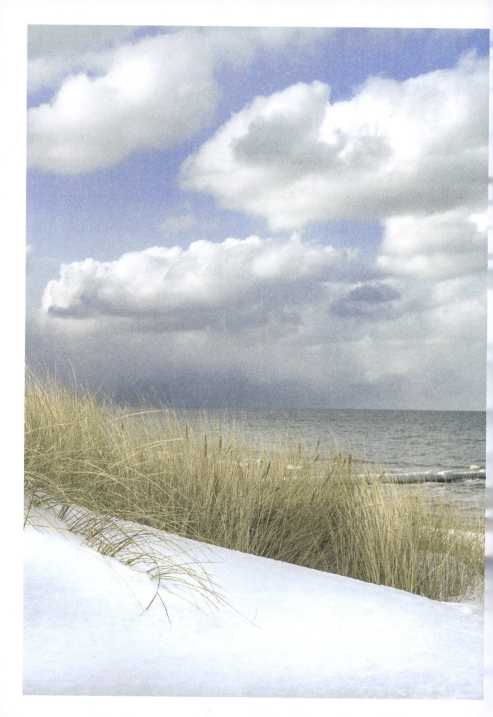

JOY FROM THE LORD

He has shown you, O mortal, what is good. And what does the LORD require of you? To act justly and to love mercy and to walk humbly with your God.
Micah 6:8

We are bombarded with advertisements at every turn. Our mailboxes are stuffed with flyers, television shows are interrupted with commercials, streaming music services blare ads every few songs, and the internet shows us all the things we don't have.

It's easy to see why we're never satisfied with what we have. We are constantly assaulted by voices that tell us we won't be happy unless we have [fill in the blank]. If we're not careful, we begin to believe these messages. But truthfully, we'll never find contentment in new clothes or the latest gadget. True contentment is found only in Christ.

Today, be mindful of the messages you believe. Every time you think, *I would be happy if I just had . . .*, ask the Lord to reveal His truth to you. You'll find rest for your soul, not by accumulating possessions but by immersing yourself in the Lord.

Dear Lord, remind me that my joy comes not from things but from You and You alone.

TO BUY OR NOT TO BUY?

*Please accept my blessing that is brought
to you, because God has dealt graciously
with me, and because I have enough.*
Genesis 33:11 ESV

One of the easiest lies to believe is that more stuff will make you happier. It's not a sin to go shopping or to buy a new car, a house, an oven, or a set of golf clubs. But if you're trying to purchase happiness and contentment, then what you are really buying is the lie.

There is nothing in this world that can perfectly satisfy. You could own a private villa in Italy, have a getaway house in the Caribbean, drive the latest model Tesla, and buy a new wardrobe every season, but without Christ, you'll never be perfectly satisfied. Only Jesus can fill the emptiness in your heart. Only He gives true contentment and joy. So if you're wondering whether to buy or not to buy, remind yourself that true contentment cannot be purchased. It can only be found in Christ. Only He will satisfy.

''''''''''''''''''''''

You are all I truly need, Jesus. Change
me until You are all I want.

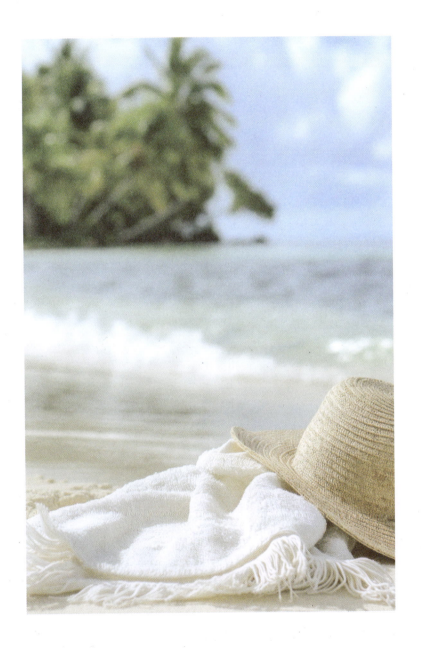

THE ULTIMATE SATISFACTION

God is able to bless you abundantly, so that in all things at all times, having all that you need, you will abound in every good work.
2 Corinthians 9:8

God will meet all your needs. Yes, all of them. In fact, *only* He can fulfill your truest and deepest needs for purpose, contentment, peace, and salvation. If dissatisfaction is stealing your rest today, you're not alone. While we live on this earth, we will deal with longing for something that seems unreachable. It's a symptom of being human. God placed a longing within us that only He can fill.

Some people turn to the stuff of this world, to others, or to jobs or hobbies for fulfillment. And while those things may temporarily bring happiness or distraction, only God can provide eternal fulfillment. He can satisfy you when nothing and no one else does. That doesn't mean you should give up all your hopes and dreams for happiness on this earth. It simply means that God has more for you, better for you, divinely perfect for you. You can rely on Him to work beyond your understanding. That's a truth you can rest in.

Lord, I know that only You can truly
satisfy; fill me with Your presence.

KNOW WHO YOU ARE

**Return to your rest, my soul, for the
Lord has been good to you.**
Psalm 116:7

There are untold numbers of products, procedures, books, and seminars that promise to make you better—more beautiful, more youthful, more confident, more financially stable. With all of that information bombarding us, we can easily become discontented with who we are.

Some days you just need to remember that you're a child of God. He created you with quirks, talents, and a one-of-a-kind personality. You are uniquely you. While it's good to work toward goals and being your best, it's also important to remember that *who you are* is enough.

When you look in the mirror today or compare yourself to someone else or wish you were somehow different, take a moment to tell yourself this: *I am enough.* God loves you simply because you are you. You don't have to become someone else in order for God to love you. Remember that you are enough, and rest in that truth today.

⁕⁕⁕⁕⁕⁕⁕⁕⁕⁕⁕⁕⁕⁕

Lord, help me find rest in knowing that You
love me simply because I am Your child.

YOU ARE A DELIGHT

**We are God's handiwork, created in
Christ Jesus to do good works, which God
prepared in advance for us to do.**
Ephesians 2:10

Y ou are an accountant, nurse, firefighter, musician. You are a father, mother, sister, grandparent, friend. You are gentle and loyal, feisty and funny, intelligent and strong. You are so many things wrapped into one body.

You are a delight, but you may not feel delightful. You may feel weak, discouraged, overwhelmed, or angry. You might even wish you were a completely different person. Maybe you want to be taller, thinner, richer, or calmer. But guess what? You're you, and there's no one else like you. You're individually made with unique gifts. Your mind, voice, laugh, and personality are wonderfully irreplaceable.

Stop trying to be someone you're not. Instead, start being the person God created you to be: yourself. Rest in that thought today, and every time you begin to criticize yourself, ask your Maker for perspective. Embrace yourself and find freedom in who you are: a beloved child of God.

When I am tempted to be someone I'm not,
remind me that I'm Your beloved child.

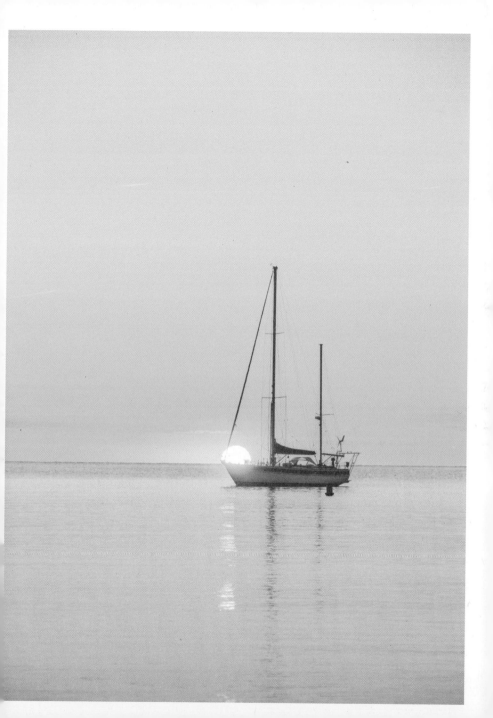

DITCHING THE PICTURE-PERFECT LIFE

What do people get for all the toil and anxious striving with which they labor under the sun?
Ecclesiastes 2:22

Social media can be fun, but it can be harmful too. If you find yourself trying to match your life to what you see online, your efforts will be futile, dear friend. Whether on Facebook, Instagram, Snapchat, or TikTok, those posts are only snapshots and sound bites of another's life. They may truly be representative of only one minute out of someone's day.

If you're trying to make your life look picture-perfect, take a rest. Instead of seeing yourself through the lens of someone else's camera, experience your life. It may be messy, broken, tear-stained, and tough. But there are also moments that make you laugh out loud and shout with joy, holy moments that remain ingrained in your mind forever. It's your life, your family, and your home—in all its glorious imperfection. Life doesn't need to be photo-worthy to be worth a great deal. Walk away from the pressure of a picture-perfect life and find rest. You'll be glad you did.

Remind me, Jesus, that this life is about loving and pleasing You today.

FIND CONTENTMENT IN YOUR STORY

O LORD, you are my God; I will exalt you; I will praise your name, for you have done wonderful things, plans formed of old, faithful and sure.
Isaiah 25:1 ESV

G od is writing a story in each of our lives. Some stories are more dramatic than others. You might have grown up in a Christian home with two loving parents, or maybe your parents divorced, leaving you dazed and wounded. Perhaps right now you are battling anxiety, or maybe you've experienced a radical transformation that brought you to Christ.

Everyone's story is different, and everyone's story is beautiful. Don't ever feel ashamed of yours. Beloved child of God, the Lord of all creation is the author of your story, and it is a reflection of His handiwork in your life. Each and every story is one of redemption and beauty.

Your story—whether it's full of drama or full of peace—has the potential to touch others' lives. Revel in the fact that God is continuing to pen your story, shaping it into a masterpiece. And because you believe in Jesus, you know it will have a happy ending.

Thank You for authoring my story, God. I find great peace in knowing You are holding the pen.

LORD, HELP ME FIND CONTENTMENT . . .

_____

_____

_____

_____

_____

_____

_____

_____

_____

_____

_____

_____

_____

_____

_____

_____

_____

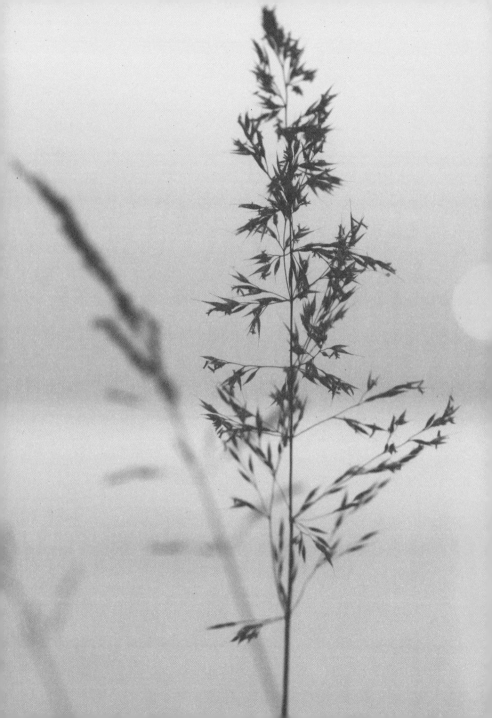

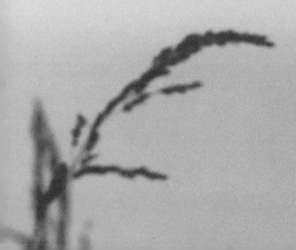

Seek Calm
in the Chaos

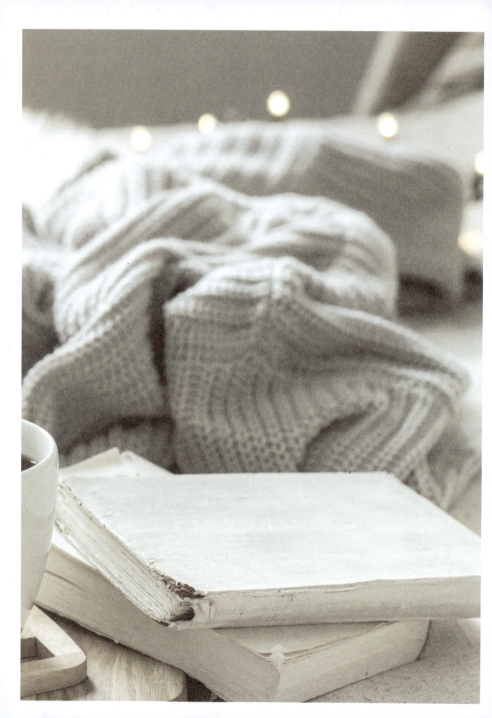

LET THE WORLD GO BY

*I have told you these things, so that in me you may
have peace. In this world you will have trouble.
But take heart! I have overcome the world.*
John 16:33

You feel frazzled. Your brain is spinning a million miles an hour, and your shoulders are so tense, they're hunched up to your ears. You have so much to do that it feels like a stretch to even sit down and read these words. Sound familiar?

Stop. For a few minutes, simply let the world pass by. Time is ticking—and it is so very valuable—but even more precious is the time you spend in rest with the Lord. Breathe deeply; calm your heart. Relax your shoulders, and let your mind become still.

Right now, in this moment, God wants you to give it all to Him: your busy schedule, your worries about finances, the stress you're feeling at work, the heartbreak you're nursing. He wants you to trust Him, and He wants you to trust that even as the world continues on, you're doing the right thing by resting in Him.

Father, help me step away from this
world's busyness and rest in You.

NO SAFER PLACE

You know the message God sent to the people of Israel, announcing the good news of peace through Jesus Christ, who is Lord of all.
Acts 10:36

The story of Jesus and His disciples caught out at sea in a storm is well known. But have you ever thought of applying that story to your own struggle for peace? Most often, we focus on Jesus' power in that story—how His simple words calmed a deadly storm. But notice what happened before He spoke: The disciples went to Jesus.

You see, the disciples were on a boat, caught in a horrendous storm. It was a matter of life or death. So what did they do? They turned to Jesus. Was their faith perfect? No. Were they still afraid? Yes. Did they doubt Him? Yes. But still they went to Him—and Jesus saved them.

Beloved, are you hurrying to Jesus when you're caught in the middle of a storm? There's no safer place. Believe in His power and strength; trust in His goodness and love. He won't let you drown.

Father, I will rest in You—especially when the storms in my life are threatening.

WHEN STORMS ROLL IN

[Jesus] awoke and rebuked the wind and said to the sea, "Peace! Be still!" And the wind ceased, and there was a great calm.
Mark 4:39 ESV

The forecast for your life looks bleak. You can see that there is pain, stress, suffering, or turmoil ahead. Your shoulders begin to hunch against the burden, and your heart races in fear. You're just not sure if you're strong enough for a storm this big.

As you watch the storm clouds rolling into your life, you might feel completely beaten. You might feel angry or sad, confused or afraid. And you may even wonder how in the world you'll get through it all. Here is your answer: Take refuge in the Lord.

Your Father in heaven might not stop the storm from coming. But He will walk through it with you. So even if the circumstances around you look treacherous, you can tell your heart, *Peace, be still*, because Jesus is with you in the boat of life. Settle into His protective arms and rest, knowing that He provides respite and refuge.

⁓⁓⁓⁓⁓⁓

You are my Rock, my Redeemer, and my Refuge,
Jesus. Thank You for Your strength in my life.

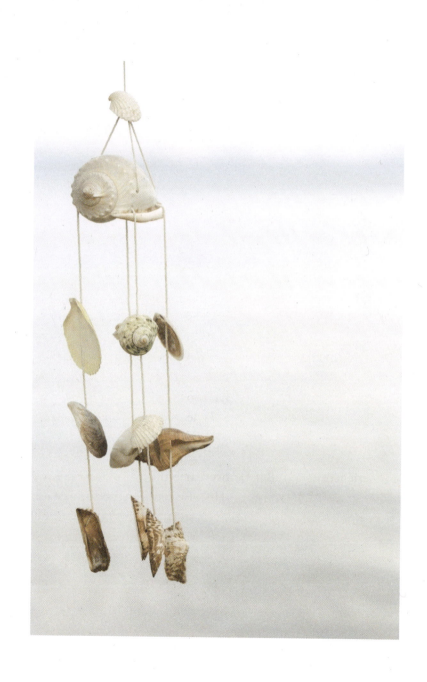

COMFORT IN A BROKEN WORLD

Even though I walk through the darkest valley,
I will fear no evil, for you are with me; your
rod and your staff, they comfort me.
Psalm 23:4

Jesus predicted that in this world we would have trouble, and the truth of that can be overwhelming at times. Our world is full of greed, ugly politics, starving families, impoverished countries, and life-threatening crime. The news headlines are often shocking and disturbing. Sometimes it seems that the world can't get any worse—but then it does.

When the world's brokenness is too much to bear, turn your eyes to Jesus. Perhaps that sounds like a cliché, but He is the only way to find comfort and peace in this broken world.

Jesus walked this earth. He understands the burden you feel because He experienced it too. But He overcame this world, and He rose up from the grave to give you eternal life. He conquered sin and death; evil doesn't get the final word. Jesus came so that we could have hope. Turn to Him, and let Him turn your sorrows into gladness, your weariness into rest.

Jesus, my heart is troubled by this world's
brokenness, but I thank You for making me whole.

KNOW MY HEART

Search me, God, and know my heart;
test me and know my anxious thoughts.
See if there is any offensive way in me,
and lead me in the way everlasting.
Psalm 139:23–24

Have you ever confessed one of your deepest, darkest secrets . . . and then waited with trepidation for a response? Hopefully, that response was filled with love and grace, for we've all fallen short of God's perfection. But if it wasn't, hear this truth: God already knows all your deepest, darkest sins, and He still loves you.

In Psalm 139 the psalmist asks God to search his heart, to know his thoughts, and to lead him. Why? Because he knows that God is a caring God who desires to make him more like Christ. While some believers may simply want God to look at their outward acts of service and compassion, the psalmist asks God to look within.

When you ask God to examine you, He'll show you how to be more pleasing to Him. He'll lead you on the right path, and He'll transform your life inside and out. He will wash you spotlessly clean of every sin. Rest in the safety and certainty of knowing that you are His own beloved child.

Lord, test me, examine me, and know my anxious
thoughts. Lead me in the way everlasting.

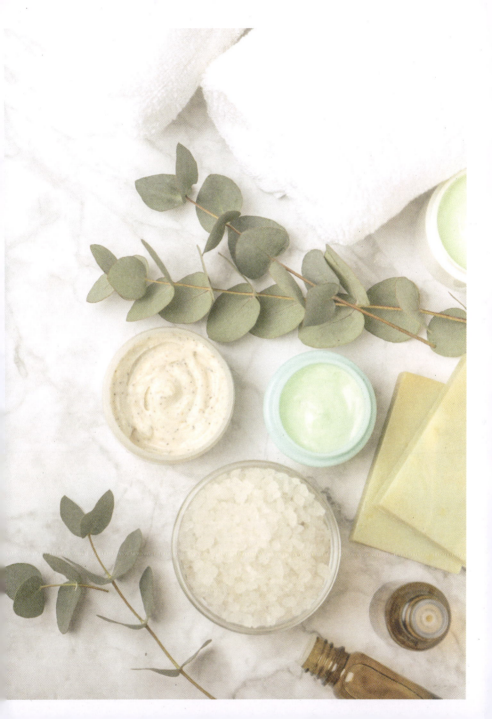

LIFE IS MESSY

I consider my life worth nothing to me; my only aim is to finish the race and complete the task the Lord Jesus has given me—the task of testifying to the good news of God's grace.
Acts 20:24

L ife is full of beautiful things: vibrant sunflowers, a perfect game, sunsets, bluebirds, and birch trees. And sometimes it's tempting to show others only the beautiful things in our lives. To present the perfect picture, we push the clutter out of the way, suck in our stomachs, throw the dishes in the dishwasher, or stash the miscellaneous piles in the spare bedroom. We don't want others to know about the messy parts.

Yes, life is beautiful, but it's also messy. And we all have our own messes—our own secrets, dirty laundry, and less-than-perfect past. The good news is this: God can turn messy into beautiful. You don't have to have it all together. It's okay if your life is less than picture-perfect.

Rely on the Lord; rest in Him. Don't hide your brokenness from Him. Not only can He mend it, but He can also transform it into something beautiful.

Father, thank You for sending Jesus to turn my messy, sinful self into something beautiful.

WORLD WEARY

**Now to him who is able to do far more abundantly
than all that we ask or think, according to
the power at work within us, to him be glory
in the church and in Christ Jesus throughout
all generations, forever and ever. Amen.**
Ephesians 3:20–21 ESV

Are you feeling world weary, dear traveler? Does it seem as if everything around you is falling apart? Are you left standing in the rubble, feeling alone and more than a little broken and bruised? Take heart—the Lord is with you.

Even in the midst of the chaos, brokenness, and trials of today, God is standing with you. In fact, He's not only standing with you, He's clearing a path for you—a path that is God-ordained and holy. You can let go of fear and worry, for the Lord is at work. All you need to do is cling to Him. There's no need to be anxious, nor do you need to despair. The Lord—incredibly mighty and Ruler of all—is close to the brokenhearted, the weary, and the troubled. You need only to be still. Breathe in His presence, for He is with you.

O Father, sometimes this world's brokenness is
too much for me. I'm so grateful You are near.

GOD CAN HANDLE THE TRUTH

If my people, who are called by my name, will humble themselves and pray and seek my face and turn from their wicked ways, then I will hear from heaven, and I will forgive their sin and will heal their land.

2 Chronicles 7:14

Have you ever done anything shameful? Are there sins you're embarrassed to tell even your closest confidant? Do you find yourself hiding from God because your failures are too shocking? Dear one, God can handle the truth.

He asks for obedience, but He welcomes the sinner. He knows no sin, but He loves those who are bound by it. God knows the darkest, most appalling parts of you, and if you confess them to Him, He will not turn you away. Instead, He will wash you clean.

If you're running from the Lord or trying to hide your mistakes, then stop. Take a deep breath and turn to Him. Know that there is nothing you can do that is beyond His forgiveness. And there is no way He can love you more or love you less than He already does. God can handle the truth, and He longs for you to stop running and, instead, find freedom in His healing presence.

Here I am, Lord, broken and sinful; thank You for loving me and covering me with Your grace.

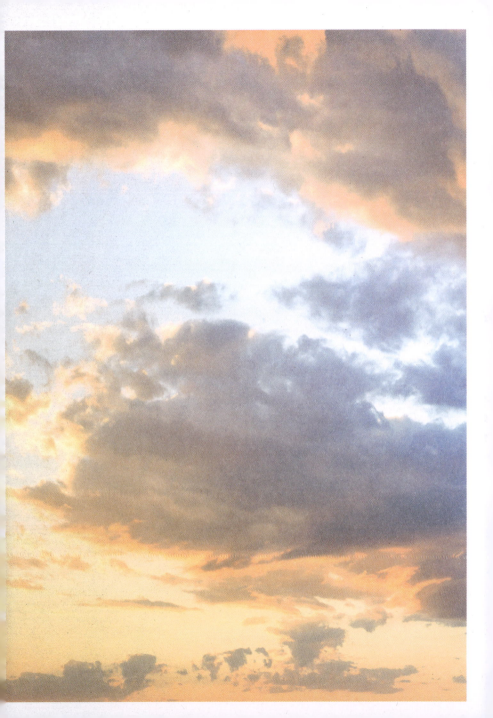

REST IN RECONCILIATION

He will yet fill your mouth with laughter
and your lips with shouts of joy.
Job 8:21

We all have difficult relationships at some point in our lives. Whether it's with our parents, siblings, fellow churchgoers, coworkers, friends, or children, relational turmoil is unavoidable. We are broken people, and we sometimes say and do hurtful things to one another.

Is there a tumultuous relationship in your life? Is it giving you anxiety or keeping you up at night? Do you have a knot in your stomach when you think about that person? If so, tell the Lord about it. Ask Him to reveal truth to your heart and the other person's heart as well.

Navigating broken relationships can be stressful, awkward, and painful. But when you are walking with the Lord, He can lift that burden from you and guide you along His perfect pathway. Ask Him to give you rest from this tough relationship today. Find comfort in knowing that He delights in walking alongside His children, even in the most difficult times.

Father, You love reconciliation. Please bring
peace to this difficult relationship.

TRUTH LIKE RAIN

*The LORD your God is with you, the Mighty
Warrior who saves. He will take great delight
in you; in his love he will no longer rebuke
you, but will rejoice over you with singing.*
Zephaniah 3:17

Y ou are God's beloved. He rejoices over you with singing and
watches over you while you sleep at night. He knit you together
with His own hands, and He delights in you. When you choose to follow
Him, He adopts you into His own family. His mercies are new every
morning, and His faithfulness continues on and on forever.

Even now, Jesus is preparing a place for you in heaven. Because of
His great and abiding love for you, He suffered, died, and rose again.
And because of His sacrifice, you are able to approach God's throne with
confidence and expectation.

When you read those words, let their truth fall on you like rain.
Let their goodness penetrate your heart and saturate your soul. You are
deeply loved by the One who formed the seas and carved the mountains. And He promises you rest from your weariness, reprieve from
your worry, and forgiveness from your sins. What a gift!

Too often I forget what a gift Your love is,
dear Lord. Thank You for loving me.

LORD, GIVE ME CALM IN THE CHAOS . . .

_____

_____

_____

_____

_____

_____

_____

_____

_____

_____

_____

_____

_____

_____

_____

_____

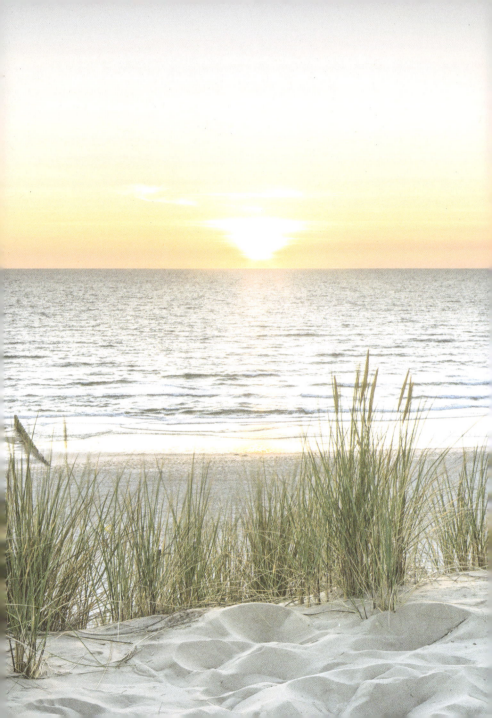

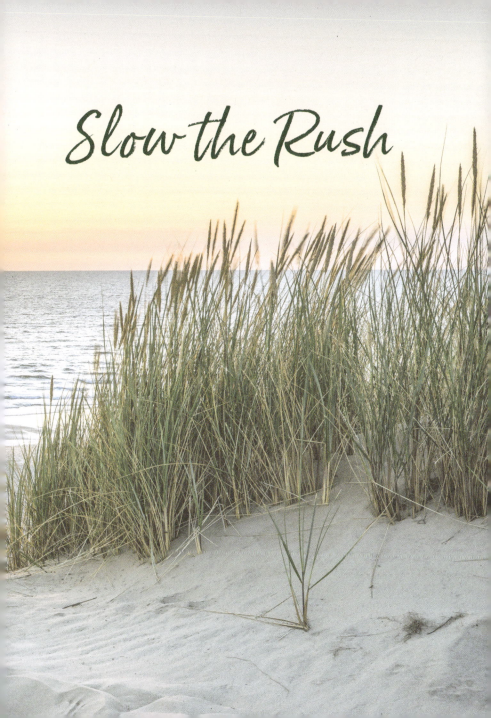

Slow the Rush

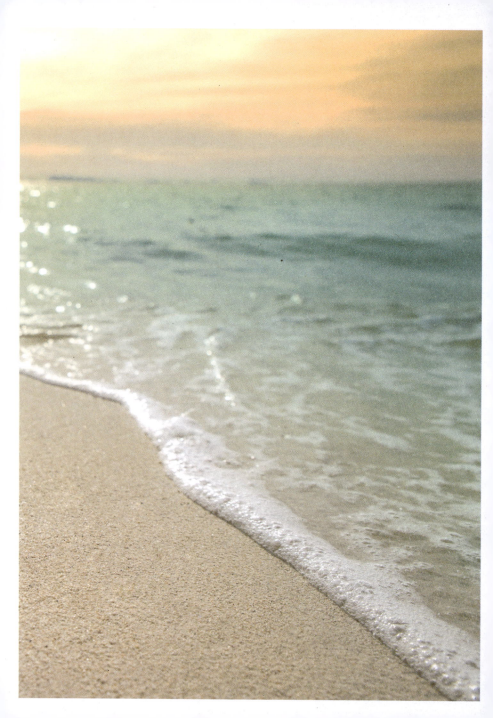

ENJOY GOD'S CREATION

**Lift up your eyes and look to the heavens:
Who created all these? He who brings out the
starry host one by one and calls forth each of
them by name. Because of his great power and
mighty strength, not one of them is missing.**
Isaiah 40:26

In today's world, children are spending more and more time inside, while experts are encouraging parents to take their kids outside. Why? Because being outside in nature helps children, not just physically but also mentally and socially. It boosts their intellect, immune system, and emotional well-being. It's just a good thing to do.

And it's not just good for children; it's good for you too. Can you find time today to go outside? Take a bike ride or get your heart rate up with a walk. Find a pool to splash in, walk by the lake, or explore a hiking trail. You'll be refreshed in a way that only the majesty of God's creation can provide. The combination of trees, fresh air, sunshine, wind, water, physical movement, the smell of dirt, and the beauty of bright blooms is healing in a unique way. So open the door and step outside. Find peace and confidence in God's creation.

The beauty of Your world amazes me, Father
God. Refresh me with Your creation.

WHEN REST SEEMS FAR AWAY

Let anyone who is thirsty come to me and drink.
John 7:37

If the word *rest* seems like a faraway, outlandish concept, these words are for you. Rest must be sought out and integrated into your life. When you aren't getting enough rest, it affects you mentally, emotionally, spiritually, and physically. But how do you fit rest into your life?

When something you need seems far away, you must begin walking toward it. Today, take one small step toward rest. It may mean saying no to something you'd normally say yes to. It may mean putting the kids to bed twenty minutes early so you can have a few minutes alone, or maybe choosing to take a five-minute walk around your office building instead of chatting by the coffee maker. Rest can come early in the morning or late at night—or even in a midafternoon reprieve with a hot cup of tea.

Over time, small steps can take you to faraway places, and rest isn't as far away as you may think.

Father, help me take one or two small
steps toward rest today.

A PATTERN OF REST

**As obedient children, do not be conformed
to the passions of your former ignorance.**
1 Peter 1:14 ESV

Romans 12:2 says, "Do not conform to the pattern of this world, but be transformed by the renewing of your mind. Then you will be able to test and approve what God's will is—his good, pleasing and perfect will." One of the patterns of our world is the pattern of busyness. The word *busy* comes out of our mouths more times than we realize; in fact, some of us can't even imagine a life that's not busy.

So when we are commanded to "not conform to the pattern of this world," it's for our own good. God wants us to conform to His example instead. Think back to the example (and command) He gave us in the Old Testament—the weekly ritual of rest.

Are you conforming to the world's pattern of busyness, or are you conforming to God's pattern of rest? Take the words of this verse to heart. Repeat them to yourself throughout the week as you seek to rest.

*I love how Your Word speaks truth to me
and guides me in my life, Father God.*

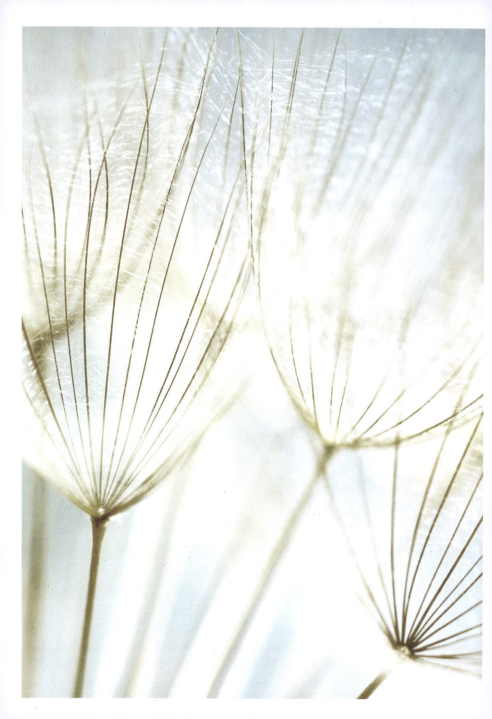

REST WITH INTENTION

Jesus withdrew again to the mountain by himself.
John 6:15 ESV

When you finally have a chance to rest, do you actually rest? Or do you fill up your free time with mindless activities such as scrolling through Instagram and refreshing your Facebook feed? When time opens up, do you see that as a chance to rest or a chance to check something off the to-do list, like shopping, cleaning, or taking on extra work?

Instead of letting precious time for yourself slip away, be intentional with it. Sit with the Lord, journal, or just let your mind relax. Do something that fills you with joy, like hiking or gardening. Times of rest need to be enjoyed, and it's only through letting yourself intentionally rest that you will feel refreshed.

Ask God for help in using your times of rest wisely. Sometimes maybe you do simply need to order pizza and watch TV. Or maybe cleaning really does de-stress and relax you. Just be sure that you are intentional during times of rest.

You gave me many examples of how to rest intentionally, Jesus. May I follow Your lead.

REST FROM OVERSCHEDULING

**The LORD replied, "My Presence will go
with you, and I will give you rest."**
Exodus 33:14

I t's a place we've all been in. You wanted a slow week, but you've overscheduled yourself. Whether you've taken on too much work, scheduled too many social outings, or said yes when you should have said no, we can all relate.

Sometimes you just have to get through an overscheduled week. Even if your commitments are set in stone, be encouraged—you can still find rest.

Whenever you take a quick time-out to eat lunch, take a shower, or drive to your next event, let your mind and body relax. Take long, deep breaths in the car. Let the hot water in your shower wash away the tension. Give thanks for your food, and take a few minutes to sit and enjoy your lunch. No, it probably won't feel as good as a two-hour nap or an afternoon at the spa, but these small moments of rest will refresh you. Wherever and whenever you can, find rest today.

⁓⁓⁓⁓⁓⁓⁓⁓⁓⁓

I feel overwhelmed today, Lord. Open up moments
of refreshment, and help me use them well.

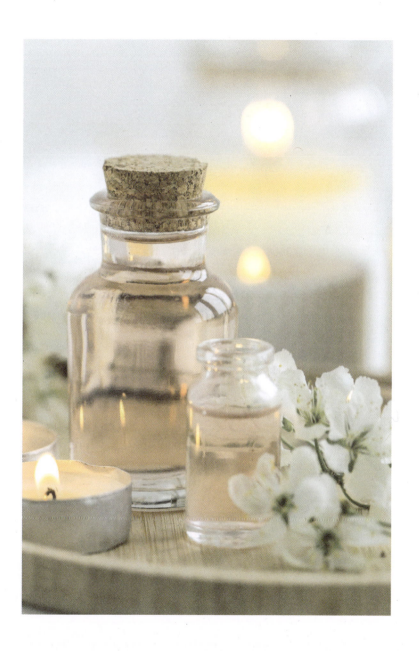

GETTING OVER OVERSCHEDULING

You, LORD, hear the desire of the afflicted; you
encourage them, and you listen to their cry.
Psalm 10:17

You look at the calendar, and your heart sinks. Every night of the week is busy, and the weekend is crammed with activities, chores, and errands. We can all relate. Overscheduling is easy to do, and it's hard to know how to maintain a less-hectic agenda. After all, the church needs you, your colleagues need you, your family needs you—and after saying yes to all their needs, there's little, if any, time left for you. Are you done with overscheduling yourself?

It's true that we all have commitments we can't bail on, and some seasons of life are busier than others. But when you're overwhelmed with overscheduling, turn to God. Give Him your schedule. Ask Him to sift through your calendar and reveal the things that can go and the things that should stay. Lean on Him and His strength. He will uphold you; He will help you; He will guide you to rest.

Lord, show me the activities I can let go of, and
guide me to those things I should keep.

WHEN WORK WORKS AGAINST YOU

The best-equipped army cannot save a king, nor is great strength enough to save a warrior.
Psalm 33:16 NLT

A strong work ethic is a great quality to have. It means you work hard and well, and you can be counted on to get the job done. But sometimes a strong work ethic can actually work against you, such as when you begin working night and day, skipping meals, and getting too little sleep because you want to do your job well.

God calls us to work hard. He wants us to work to the best of our ability and to honor and glorify His name through our efforts. But He doesn't want to see us burned out, struggling to stay awake, or becoming resentful of our jobs.

Does your work ethic work against you? Admit that you can't do it all—because you weren't created to do it all. Then treat yourself to some rest. Take a Sabbath; go on a weekend trip. God worked, and then He rested. Take some time to follow His example.

I admit that I can't do it all, Lord.
Rescue me with Your rest.

NO GUILT IN NO

All you need to say is simply "Yes" or "No."
Matthew 5:37

Fact: When you say no to one thing, it allows you to say yes to other things that are more important to you.

If you're a people pleaser, it's difficult to say no. You'd rather say yes and overwhelm yourself than say no and disappoint someone else. But when your yeses begin to pile up, they take valuable time away from other aspects of your life: your work, friends, family, church life, and your rest. Of course it feels good to help someone out. But sometimes you're hurting yourself in the process.

That's why guilt shouldn't be attached to the word *no.* Saying no isn't selfish or self-centered or greedy; it's simply treating your own time as valuable. Jesus didn't say yes to everyone; He left the crowds, spent time with His disciples, and rested.

If you catch yourself saying yes out of guilt today, stop and ask God if you should—politely, gently, and lovingly—say no.

When I begin to say yes out of guilt, Lord,
stop me and remind me of my limits.

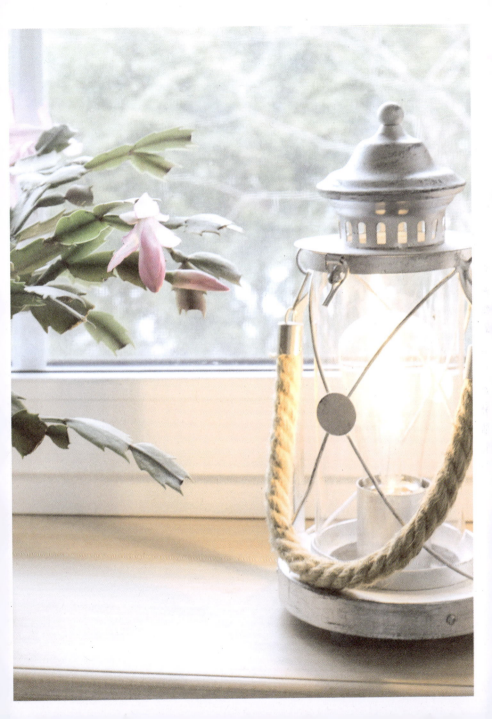

FIGHT THE RUSH

Be joyful in hope, patient in affliction, faithful in prayer.
Romans 12:12

Rushing has become the norm in today's culture. We rush from meeting to meeting, incessantly checking our email in between. We rush the kids to school, to doctor's appointments, and to after-school activities. We rush home to dinner and time with the family, or we rush to a dinner date with friends, out of breath and five minutes late.

What would your life look like without rushing? It's not easy to slow down, but it's possible. It must be done with intention and reliance on God, because living life at a slower pace doesn't come naturally. With practice, however, it can begin to feel natural.

How can you slow down today? Give yourself five more minutes to eat breakfast; taste the food instead of shoveling it down. Leave work early enough to beat rush-hour traffic and arrive home relaxed rather than tense. Choose one way to slow down today—and take a rest from the rush.

Instead of rushing and stress, please give me stillness and peace, Father God.

EYES WIDE OPEN

**Sing to him, sing praise to him; tell
of all his wonderful acts.**
1 Chronicles 16:9

If you've ever taken a walk with a young child, you know it's often more stopping than walking. She'll want to look at every bug, crack in the sidewalk, fallen leaf, and budding flower. He'll bend down to inspect a colony of ants and look up to see the airplane roaring overhead. Children live with their eyes wide open.

Unfortunately, as we grow into adults, something changes. Pebbles and grass are exchanged for phones and laptop screens. That sense of wonder is replaced with worry and stress. Instead of taking our time, we rush, rush, rush. We don't stop to see the beauty around us.

Slow down and keep your eyes wide open. Notice the way your spouse laughs or your dog settles in the sunlight. Breathe in the aroma of fresh bread as you pass the bakery. Savor your cup of coffee. Living with eyes wide open will invite more wonder into your life—and a more restful, childlike spirit.

*Jesus, help me recapture my wonder
for You, Your earth, and my life.*

LORD, HELP ME SLOW THE RUSH ...

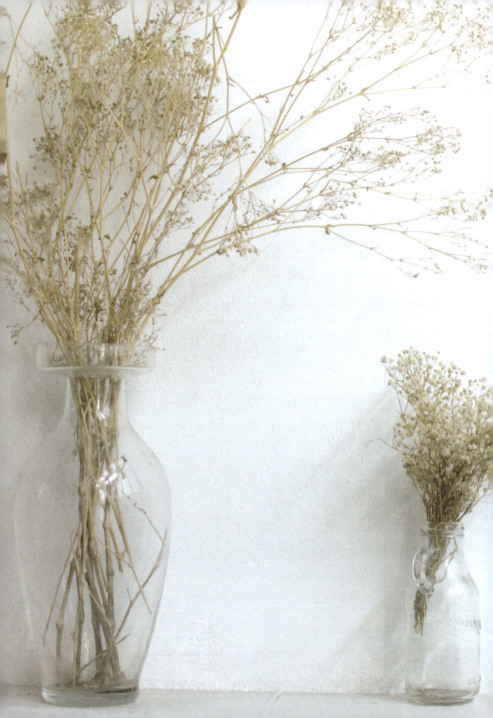

Quiet Your Soul

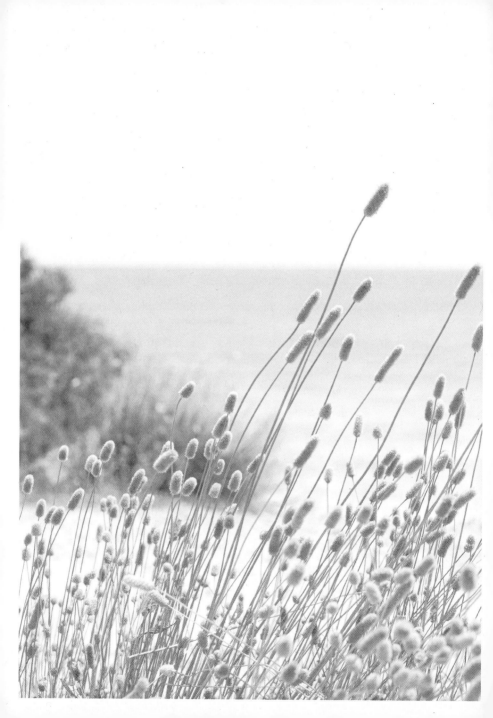

RESTORE AND RENEW

For the sake of my family and friends,
I will say, "Peace be within you."
Psalm 122:8

When Jesus drew away from the crowds and found a place alone to pray, He was resting with His Father. He did it on purpose and with intention. How often do you find yourself resting intentionally and on purpose? And no, falling asleep on the couch doesn't count! Only intentional rest brings true restoration.

You have permission to intentionally rest today, friend. Sit with a cup of coffee for a few extra minutes. Take some time for an afternoon stroll through the park. Put aside your responsibilities this evening and enjoy some quality time with your spouse instead.

Continual work will leave you worn out and empty, but purposefully seeking out rest will bless you with restoration and renewal for your soul.

Restore my soul and renew my body.
Father, please draw near to me.

GIVE YOURSELF GRACE

**The Lord make his face shine on you and
be gracious to you; the Lord turn his
face toward you and give you peace.**
Numbers 6:25–26

We are our own worst critics. Whether you mess up during a work presentation or yell at your children or put your foot in your mouth yet again, you're most often the only one beating yourself up afterward. Dear friend, give yourself a little grace.

You don't need to keep replaying your mistakes or reliving your bad moments. You can find comfort in the Savior who washes you clean, over and over. He does not hold resentment toward you. Breathe deep in the knowledge that you are loved—flaws and all. Revel in the fact that you are covered with grace. And when you begin chastising yourself, when those words of self-condemnation ring in your ears, try to see yourself through the eyes of your loving Father.

Give yourself grace, resting in the knowledge that He removes all your sins from you gladly and willingly.

Lord, Your forgiveness knows no bounds.
Teach me to give myself grace.

YOU ARE UNIQUE

So God created human beings in his own image. In the image of God he created them; male and female he created them.
Genesis 1:27 NLT

What is your favorite thing about yourself? Is it your unique laugh or the color of your eyes? Is it your contagious love for others or your mathematical mind? Maybe you love your ability to run or your quiet confidence. There are many things to love about yourself—after all, you were created in the image of a perfect God!

There are also things that make you unique—things that you may not be quite so fond of. Do you have funny-shaped feet or a tendency to turn bright red when embarrassed? Do you carry the family nose or cry at the drop of a hat? Your uniqueness isn't bad, and it doesn't need to be fixed.

Stop trying to hide or change those unique things about you. They form who you are, and you are beloved by God. Rest in accepting your individuality today.

Father, help me rest in my uniqueness. Teach me to take pleasure in the quirks that make me, me!

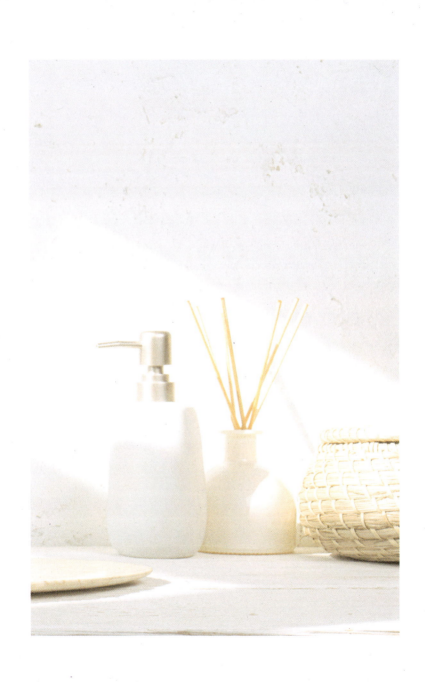

THE WORDS OF MY MOUTH

May these words of my mouth and this meditation of my heart be pleasing in your sight, Lord, my Rock and my Redeemer.
Psalm 19:14

Your words have power. Not only the power to impact someone else but also the power to alter your own thinking. Ponder this: If your words are always full of complaints about life's busyness and difficulties, you're going to believe that life is negative.

Why not try a different way? Instead of distress, speak words of hope in the Lord and joy in His faithfulness. When you remind yourself of these truths, you'll begin believing them and acting on them—and filling your life with positivity and praise.

When negative words spring to your lips, try giving thanks to the Lord instead. When despair creeps into your conversation, declare the truths of who God is and what He says in His Word. The Lord brings light, not darkness; He brings peace, not strife; and He offers hope, not despair. Rest in the power of praising Him.

May the words of my mouth always be pleasing to You, Lord.

SIT AND LISTEN

If my people would only listen to me.
Psalm 81:13

There are many different ideas of what your time with God should look like: intensive Bible study with concordances and commentaries, journaling, quiet reflection, a daily devotional, a walk in the woods. Yes, there are countless ways to spend time with the Lord, and one of those is rest.

What if you simply sat quietly in His presence and listened? What if you brought nothing to your quiet time except a listening ear and an open heart? It may be a foreign concept to you, and you might even feel as if you're doing something wrong by not doing anything. But sometimes we need to sit in the Lord's presence and open our hearts to Him. Allow yourself to find rest in the open arms of a perfect, loving, and holy God; sometimes that's just what you need.

Today, look to your heavenly Father and simply relish knowing that He loves you and that He is with you and for you.

Father, my heart is open and listening to hear Your voice. Thank You for speaking to Your child.

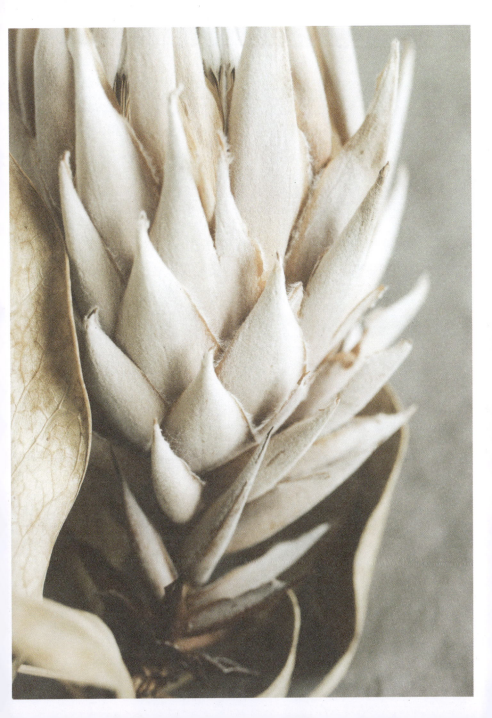

PEACE FROM WITHIN

You are my strength, I sing praise to you; you, God,
are my fortress, my God on whom I can rely.
Psalm 59:17

Have you ever met someone who had an unbelievably crazy-busy schedule, but instead of being stressed and fatigued, they exuded a peaceful calm and an utter reliance on Jesus? That's called inner rest. It's a peace that depends not upon circumstances, personality, or even organization; instead, it comes from a prayerful spirit and an intentional dependence on the Lord.

With inner rest, your life may look hectic on the outside, and you may not get as much sleep as you'd like each night, but your daily, hourly, and sometimes minute-by-minute surrendering to the Lord keeps your spirit firmly planted in peace instead of despair.

Dear friend, do you need internal rest today? It's available to you. Ask the Lord to lead you to true, deep, inner rest, to the peace and calm that can only come from Him. Ask, and He will give you rest.

O God, I deeply desire inner rest. Please help
me surrender my life completely to You.

TURN DOWN THE NOISE

*The LORD is in his holy temple; let all
the earth be silent before him.*
Habakkuk 2:20

F inding a quiet place may sound simple to do, but it rarely is in this noise-filled world. It's easy to get caught up in the hustle, bustle, speed, and anxiety of life. Sitting in a quiet place to rest for a bit almost feels . . . wasteful and decadent. But, dear friend, that's just what you need to do.

Turning down the noise and tuning out everything except the voice of your heavenly Father is crucial. Sitting with Him in the morning, at the end of the day, or any time at all will calm your soul. Just a few moments of silence in His presence will help refocus your eyes and heart on Him instead of on yourself and your own strength. Let His voice speak over any troubles you have in your life and allow the quiet power of His Word to penetrate your soul. Let God give you rest.

Father, help me tune out the noise of
the world and focus on You.

SIT STILL

**The eyes of the LORD are everywhere, keeping
watch on the wicked and the good.**
Proverbs 15:3

A s you read these words, do you feel the urge to get up and do something? Are you comfortable sitting still, or do you feel a bit of guilt about even taking time to read this?

We all need time to simply be still, so let yourself sit. God wants to speak to you, and He often speaks loudest when you push away distractions, stop working, and open your ears to what He has to say. Sitting still may feel lazy or unnatural; it might take everything you have not to scroll through your phone or check your email. But being in the Lord's presence may actually be the most productive part of your whole day.

Start your morning with the Giver of life. Let Him carry you and speak to you. Your mindset and attitude are changed in the presence of Holy God—and all you need to do is be still and listen.

*My ears are open, my body is still, and my spirit
is ready. Speak to Me, precious Jesus.*

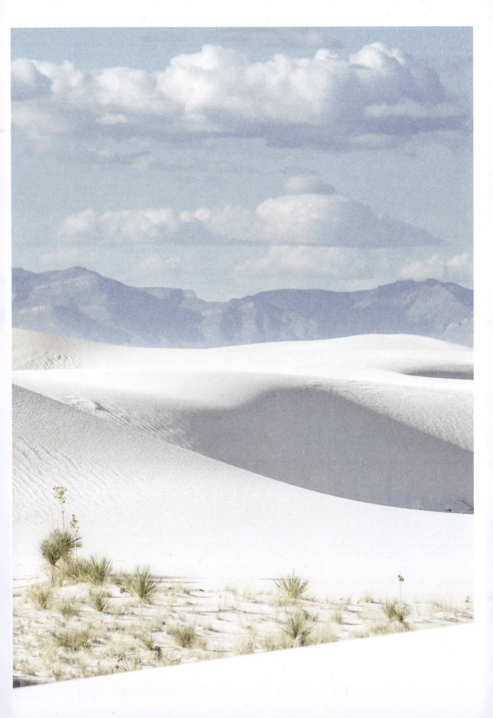

THE GIFT OF SILENCE

**It is good to wait quietly for the
salvation of the Lord.**
Lamentations 3:26

Our world is loud. It's busy. It's fast. Silence is a stranger that, so often, we run away from. We insert our earbuds and navigate to the latest music-streaming service or podcast. We lose ourselves in TikTok or YouTube. But how often do we let our world go silent?

When we rush through our days and weeks in a roar of constant noise, God's still, small voice tends to get muffled. We stop listening for Him and instead listen to the loudest voices and turn to the most pressing priorities. We can't hear God's voice when we're filling our ears with everything else.

Dear friend, embrace the silence. Sit in quiet stillness with the Lord today. It might be uncomfortable—you might even feel jittery at first. You'll probably feel the urge to fidget or scroll through your phone or check the news. But it's in the quiet that God's still, small voice is best heard. Silence the noise and find rest in listening to Him.

Here I am, Lord. I'm stepping away from
the noise and listening for Your voice.

WELCOME SILENCE

Tremble and do not sin; when you are on your beds, search your hearts and be silent.
Psalm 4:4

I n today's world, it's so easy to busy ourselves with distractions. We can turn to our phones, click the remote, put in some headphones, or turn on the computer. There is so much we can—and often do—turn to in order to fill the silence. But silence can be your place of rest.

Certainly, it can be almost frightening to let your world become still. It might even seem easier to quiet your worries or insecurities with a funny sitcom or a Facebook binge. But what would happen if you simply sat? If you welcomed silence?

Thankfully, our God doesn't choose to distract Himself from our troubles. Instead, He faces them head-on and promises to come to our defense. "The LORD will fight for you; you need only to be still" (Exodus 14:14). Sit in silence and stillness with the Lord today. Don't mute your fears with the noise of distraction; let Him fight for you.

Lord Jesus, You are my strength and help in times of need. With You, I can face my fears.

LORD, HELP ME QUIET MY SOUL . . .

_____

_____

_____

_____

_____

_____

_____

_____

_____

_____

_____

_____

_____

_____

_____

_____

_____

_____

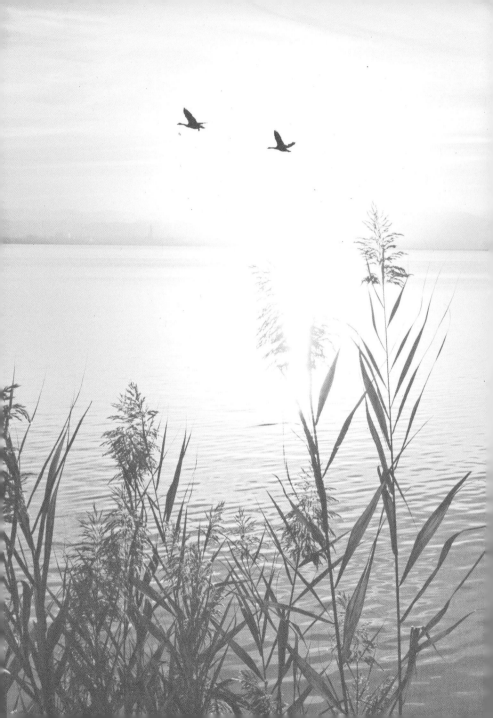

Rest in the Lord

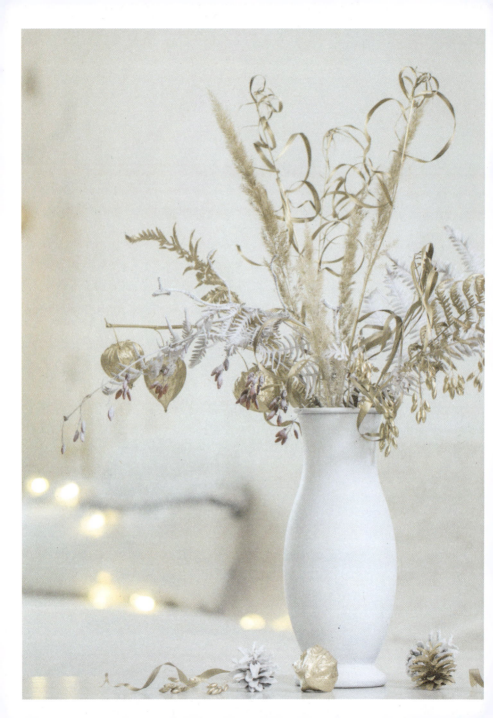

LEAVE IT AT THE CROSS

He himself bore our sins in his body on the tree,
that we might die to sin and live to righteousness.
By his wounds you have been healed.
1 Peter 2:24 ESV

What's weighing heavily on your mind today? Is it the sin that so easily entangles you? Are you waiting for the doctor to reveal test results? Are you worried about your son or daughter, your parents, or your partner? Do you feel as if you're in over your head? Maybe you feel unloved and unwanted. Whatever it is, it's not too heavy for the cross.

Write down your burdens today—all of them. Whether you're worried about your sickly dog, the paper you need to write, the continuous car repairs, or your grandmother's cancer, write it down. Then picture yourself taking this list of burdens and worries to the cross.

Jesus will take that list from you. He wants to carry your burdens for you. He wants to relieve you of the fears you're holding on to and the shame you may be feeling. He wants you to take everything to the cross—and leave it there.

Father, thank You for bearing my burdens.
Remind me to leave them with You.

A PAUSE ON PLEASING

**The Lord looks down from heaven on
all mankind to see if there are any who
are wise, who want to please God.**
Psalm 14:2 TLB

I am disappointed in you. I was counting on you. I needed you, and you weren't there. Those are hard words to hear. Some people so dread disappointing others that they strive to please everyone all the time. They work and work and then work some more to make sure everyone is happy.

But trying to please everyone is exhausting and impossible. Admit it—you can't make everyone happy. Of course, you can say yes to some things, but it's not your duty to say yes to all things. Sometimes you simply need to say no to others and yes to God and yourself. Putting God first and giving some priority to nourishing your own body and soul are actually key components in being able to serve others well.

Do you need to put a pause on pleasing others today? Ask the Lord to help you put pleasing Him at the top of your to-do list.

*Jesus, help me establish healthy boundaries and
remind me to focus on You first and foremost.*

PERFECT TIMING

*Oh, the depth of the riches of the wisdom
and knowledge of God! How unsearchable his
judgments, and his paths beyond tracing out!*
Romans 11:33

Dear friend, are you learning the hard truth that God's timing is not your own? Are you anxious to see your prayers answered? Are you frustrated that nothing is happening the way you thought it should? Don't worry—you are not alone. We have all struggled with understanding God's timing at one point or another, but here's the reassuring truth: God is in control. He loves you as His own child, and He'll always do what is ultimately best for you.

Just as a father loves to give good gifts to his children, the Lord loves to bless you. You can rest in His plans because He is your loving and generous Father, because He'll be with you every step of the way, and because His plans are better than any plan you could devise for yourself. Let go of the reins and rest instead in God's promises, plans, and perfect timing.

Father, I believe Your plans are better than
my own. Help me see that truth.

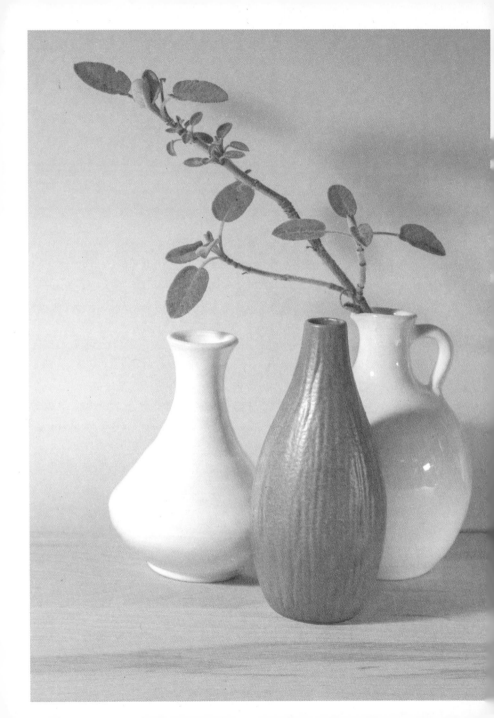

THE LORD IS NEAR

**I tell you, whatever you ask for in prayer, believe
that you have received it, and it will be yours.**
Mark 11:24

If you read through the book of Psalms, you'll know that David
endured moments of great pain in his life. Many times, he cried out
to God in despair, wept with sorrow, and begged God to come to his aid
and defeat his enemies.

Maybe you're feeling a whole lot of pain right now. Your heart is
broken, and the circumstances you're in feel bleak. Perhaps it's physical
pain you're battling or maybe the loss of a loved one. Do you feel lonely?
Do you feel sad? Turn your eyes to heaven; the Lord is near.

Do as David did; call upon the Lord continually. Open your heart to
Him. God doesn't need wordy, poetic prayers; simple and open honesty
is all He seeks. And you don't have to have everything figured out—
that's what God is there for. Just call out to Him in your pain, believe in
Him, trust Him, and He will give you peace.

O Lord my God, I cry out to You.
Rescue me and give me peace.

REJECTION HAPPENS

**There is now no condemnation for those who
are in Christ Jesus, because through Christ
Jesus the law of the Spirit who gives life has
set you free from the law of sin and death.**

Romans 8:1–2

We all want to be loved, to be admired, and to receive applause for our successes. We want to have friends and relationships and nods of approval from many. We don't want to be rejected.

But because we are broken people, rejection will inevitably rear its head. Your boss might not recommend you for the promotion; a budding friendship might turn ugly; you might be left out, uninvited. Rejection happens, and it hurts. You might wonder if you should even keep trying, or if you should just sit back and let life happen. Fear of rejection is real.

Are you struggling with that fear today? If so, rest in these words from Jesus: "There is no judgment against anyone who believes in him" (John 3:18 NLT). The Lord won't reject you; He is a safe place to rest.

Father, rejection makes me want to run and
hide. Thank You for never rejecting me.

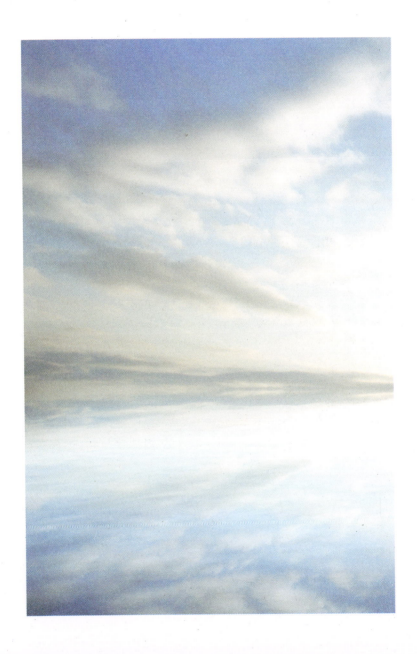

REST IN GRACE

**All have sinned and fall short of the glory of God,
and are justified by his grace as a gift, through
the redemption that is in Christ Jesus.**
Romans 3:23–24 ESV

Ephesians 2:8 says, "For by grace you have been saved through faith. And this is not your own doing; it is the gift of God" (ESV). Did you see that, dear reader? You are not saved through your own works. God isn't counting the number of times you do something good, and He isn't waiting for you to reach a magic number to give you salvation. He isn't looking at you to save yourself; salvation is His gift.

You are saved by grace, and it is only by grace that you can come before the Lord. It is only because of God's grace that you can have eternal life. It has nothing to do with what you do—it's all about what Christ did.

Isn't that a life-changing gift? We can rest in the salvation of Christ. We do not have to work for God's love; it's already ours. Praise the Lord, for He has done good things for us!

*Your grace brings me to my knees and humbles
me. Thank You, Lord, thank You!*

THE SUN WILL RISE

May our Lord Jesus Christ himself and God our Father . . . encourage your hearts and strengthen you in every good deed and word.
2 Thessalonians 2:16–17

When the sun sets, and you fall into bed after a particularly rough day, do you ever feel as if the whole world is against you? Your kids are demanding, your work is stressing you out, your responsibilities are overwhelming, and everything would be so much better if you just had a little more time. Sound familiar?

Remember, my friend, that after every bad night there is a new sunrise, every frustrating day can be followed by a joyful evening, and each bad start can end with a fantastic finish. When God says His mercies are new every morning, He means it. He has more than enough grace for you each day. You can be sure of it—as sure as the sun rises. Find peace today in knowing that God gives you new beginnings . . . over and over and over again.

Thank You, Jesus, for Your grace upon grace—in the morning, in the evening, and every moment in between.

WHEN LIFE IS PAINFUL

How long, O LORD? Will you forget me forever?
How long will you hide your face from me? . . . But
I have trusted in your steadfast love; my heart
shall rejoice in your salvation. I will sing to the
LORD, because he has dealt bountifully with me.
Psalm 13:1, 5–6 ESV

The psalmist David made lots of mistakes and suffered the consequences. He often felt far from God, and at times he even despaired.

Are you going through a painful time in your life? Is your heart broken into so many pieces that you wonder if it will ever be whole again? You may be suffering physical pain, or perhaps you've lost a loved one. Maybe you are experiencing depression, or you feel a deep loneliness. There are many ways pain can appear in our lives, and it can feel like an impossible burden. Take heart, dear one, for when life is painful, the Lord is right beside you.

God isn't far away, up in the sky, ignoring you. No, He is bearing the pain right along with you. He is wrapping His arms around you and shedding tears with you. Cry out to Him and find rest in His comfort and strength.

How long, O Lord, will I feel this pain?
Lift it away and dry my tears.

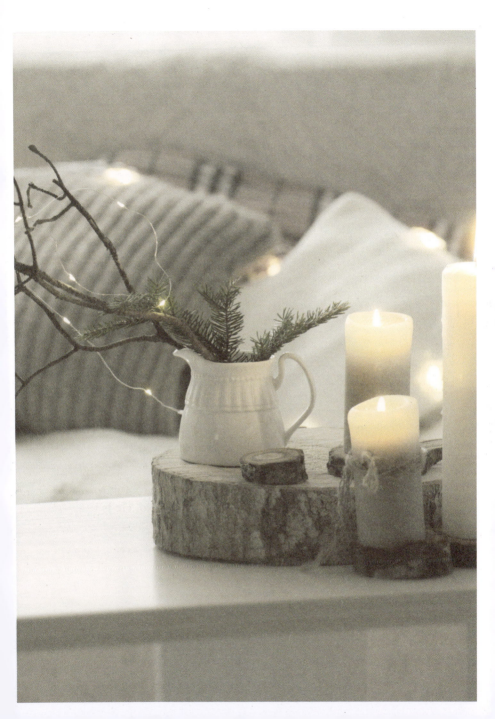

THE BEST VERSION
OF YOURSELF

**For the foolishness of God is wiser than
human wisdom, and the weakness of God
is stronger than human strength.**
1 Corinthians 1:25

want to be a better parent." "I want to have a better job." "I want to
get better grades." "I want to be a more loving son."

There are so many ways we can better ourselves, and as Christians,
we should try to be the best we can be. We need to do our best to be a
good mother or father, neighbor or friend, sister or brother, colleague
or boss. And yes, we need to do all things as if we're doing them for
God. But we should also acknowledge this truth: We can't be the best
at everything.

Do you ever feel overwhelmed by the things you need or want to
excel at? Bring these concerns to the Lord. He knows exactly what you
need, and He can help you see what is truly important. And He can
gently, patiently, and tenderly transform you into the best version of
yourself. Trust Him.

I want to be transformed, Lord, but
I need Your help to do it.

JESUS, OUR FRIEND

If anyone is in Christ, the new creation has come: The old has gone, the new is here!
2 Corinthians 5:17

Do you have a friend who's never uttered a bad word about you? One who would do anything for you without blinking an eye? Have you ever had a friend who always speaks lovingly, patiently, and wisely, and who has never, ever sinned? Your friends may have many wonderful, positive traits, but all have sinned and fallen short of perfection. All except Jesus.

Jesus is the perfect Friend. He'll never stab you in the back. He'll never spread gossip about you or use you to get ahead. He'll never belittle you or snap at you in anger. He'll never disappoint you. But He will always love you.

Jesus' friendship gives rest to wandering and hungry souls. You don't need to earn His love; you can rest fully knowing that He loves you unconditionally and perfectly. What a Friend you have in Jesus!

*Your love and mercy bring me to my knees,
Jesus. Thank You for being my Friend.*

LORD, HELP ME REST IN YOU ...

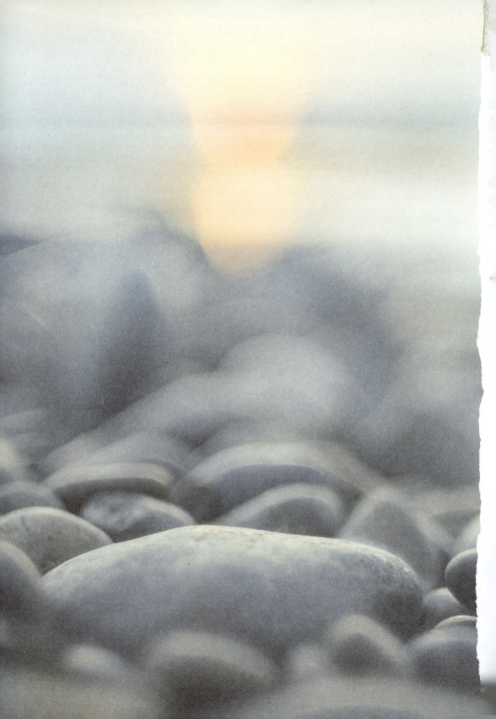